MEDICAL
TERMINOLOGY

A Quick & Easy Reference Book:
The Basics of Terminology, Anatomy, and Abbreviations

G. CHEN, MS, PHD &
STEPHEN LEESBURG

Medical Terminology, A Quick & Easy Reference Book: The Basics of Terminology, Anatomy, and Abbreviations, 3rd Edition

Library of Congress Cataloging-in-Publication Data

Names: Chen, G., author. | Leesburg, Stephen, author.
Title: Medical Terminology, A Quick & Easy Reference Book:
The Basics of Terminology, Anatomy, and Abbreviations/
G. Chen, Stephen Leesburg
Description: Third edition. | Lancaster, Pennsylvania:
PENN Medical Education Publishing, 2023
Identifiers: LCCN 2023904933 | ISBN 9781950159581
Subjects: | MESH: Medicine | Terminology
Classification: LCC R123 | NLM W 15 | DDC 610.1/4--dc23
LC record available at https://lccn.loc.gov/2023904933

Library of Congress Control Number: 2023904933
ISBN: 978-1-950159-58-1

Printed in the United States of America.

TABLE OF CONTENTS

INTRODUCTION

Whether looking for a refresher on medical terminology, an occasional reference tool, or a way to get started with studying for your respective field in medicine, you'll find this book indispensable. First, though, here are a few words about what to expect, so you know what this book is and isn't.

For everyone, you'll notice that affixes appear multiple times throughout the book. That's on purpose! The idea is to provide a quick and easy reference in any instance. For example, if you encounter a word without context and need to better understand the meaning, you can flip to the alphabetical section and quickly find any prefix, root word, or suffix needed.

Or let's say you're struggling to recall a certain word related to a specific bodily system. In this book, you can simply flip to the section on that system to (most likely) find the answer.

If you're just getting started and have not yet learned medical terminology, you'll probably want to start at the beginning. Get familiar with the basics and take your time. This book is not, in and of itself, a "study guide." And while you won't find any "quizzes," the book design includes the affixes of words in cleanly delineated tables so that, if you wish, you can cover up part of the page with a sheet and quiz yourself as you scroll through the tables.

Lastly, this book is not meant to be a comprehensive anatomy reference guide. Again, however, for quick reference for those who need it, we do cover some of the basics for major body systems, body cavities, and so forth. While this information could help those still in the early stages of learning gross anatomy, the details are meant merely as a reference to put some of the terminology into context and should not be used as a comprehensive anatomical guide. That kind of book exists, of course, but it's a different kind of reference altogether.

BASICS OF TERMINOLOGY: ROOTS, SUFFIXES, AND PREFIXES

Many words are, in and of themselves, little stories, meaning they have a beginning, middle, and end. These parts are the prefix, the root word, and the suffix, respectively.

Not all words have all three parts. Sometimes a word has just the prefix and root, sometimes just the root and suffix, and sometimes multiple roots. But importantly, a word is never made up *only* of prefixes or suffixes. Every word has at least one root word, or main idea.

For example, let's look at the word *reviewing*. It means *viewing something again*. Here are the parts of the word:

Prefix = re

Root = view

Suffix = ing

Re is a prefix that basically means *again*.

View is a root word that means *see* or *look*.

-ing is a suffix implying the root word is occurring. When reviewing, you're viewing something again.

Thus, the root word conveys the main idea (i.e., view).

Let's get concrete: If you approached a friend and just said "again," you'd proba- bly get a funny look and a response something like "What again?" Similarly, if you just said "doing," your friend would likely say something like "Doing what?"

If you just said "look," your friend would try to see where you're looking to deter- mine what you're seeing. Your friend may not know what to look for, but the idea behind your words is clear. If you run into a word you don't know, first ask your- self this question: "What is the what?"

Here's another example: *unemployment*

Prefix = un

Root = employ

Suffix = ment

You can't just say "un" or "ment" and expect to be understood, but when you add the main idea, *employ,* the word makes sense. It means the *state of not having a job*.

Where Things Gets Messy

Of course, we speak the English language—a marvelous but maddening amalga- mation of many other languages, mostly Latin, German, and Greek. That means many root words are not English words. On top of that, no hard-and-fast rules exist for how prefixes and suffixes will change root words, so each root may look a little different depending on which prefixes and suffixes are used.

However, you can usually get the gist by first breaking off the parts that you know are prefixes and suffixes and then asking yourself what the remaining part reminds you of.

To break things down correctly, though, you need to have a grasp of the most common prefixes, suffixes, and root words. The subsections below give you some examples of the most common ones in all three categories.

Common English Prefixes

Below are some common *opposite* prefixes:

Prefix	Variations	Meaning	Examples
Anti-	Ant-	against or opposite	anti-inflammatory, antagonist
De-		opposite	decontaminate, deconstruct
Dis-		not or opposite	disagree, dis (slang for insult)
In-	Im-, Ii-, Ir-	not	incapable, impossible, illegitimate, irreplaceable
Non-		not	noncompliant, nonsense
Un-		not	unfair, unjust

Below is a quick list of some additional common prefixes:

Prefix	Variations	Meaning	Examples
En-	Em-	cause	enlighten, empower
Fore-		before	foresee, foretell
In-		inside of	inland, income
Inter-		between	interrupt, interaction
Mid-		in the middle of	midair, midlife
Mis-		wrong	mistake, misdiagnose
Pre-		before	pregame, prefix
Re-		again	review, recompress
Semi-		half or partial	semitruck, semiannual
Sub-		under	subconscious, subpar
Super-		above	superimpose, superstar
Trans-		across	translate, transform

Common English Suffixes

Suffix	Variations	Meaning	Examples
-able	-ible	can be accomplished	capable, possible
-al	-lal	has the traits of	additional, beneficial
-en		made of	molten, wooden
-er		more than	luckier, richer
-er	-or	agent that does	mover, actor
-est		most	largest, happiest
-ic		has the traits of	acidic, dynamic
-ing		continues to do	reviewing, happening
-ion	-tion, -ation, -ition	process of	occasion, motion, rotation, condition
-ity		the state of	ability, simplicity
-ly		has the traits of	friendly, kindly
-ment		process/state of	enlightenment, establishment
-ness		state of	happiness, easiness
-ous	-eous, -lous	has the traits of	porous, gaseous, conscious
-y		has the traits of	artsy, classy

Common Root Words

If you can't identify a word because it seems like it's in another language, that's most likely because the word *is* in another language. This isn't always true, of course, but a good general rule is that longer, more academic English words tend to have their roots in Latin and Greek, while shorter English words tend to have their roots in German. For example, *amorous* and *loving* are synonyms, but one has its roots in the Latin *amor* and the other in the German *lieb*, respectively.

Latin/Greek Roots

Below are some of the common, yet longer and more academic Latin and Greek roots:

Root	Variations	Meaning	Examples
Andro		male or man	astronomy, disaster
Aqua		water	aquatic, aquarium
Aud		hear	auditorium, audience
Bene	Ben	good	benevolent, benign
Bio		life	biology, autobiography
Cent		hundred	century, cent (money)
Chrono		time	chronological, synchronize
Circum	Circa	around	circumspect, circumnavigate, circadian
Contra	Counter	against or conflict	contraband, encounter
Diet		speak or say	dictate, dictation
Duc	Duct, duce	lead or leader	produce, conduct
Fac		make or do	manufacture, facsimile (fax)
Fract	Frag	break	fraction, defragment
Gen		birth or create	genetics, generate
Graph		write	telegraph, calligraphy
Ject		throw	inject, projection
Jur	Jus	law	juror, justice
Log	Logue	concept or thought	logo, dialogue
Mal		bad	maladaptive, malevolent

(Continued)

Root	Variations	Meaning	Examples
Man		hand	manuscript, manual
Mater		mother	maternal, material
Mis	Mit	send	mission, submit
Pater	Pat	father	paternal, patriot
Path		feel	sympathy, empathetic
Phile	Philo	love	philosophy, anglophile
Phon		sound	telephone, phonetic
Photo		light	photograph, photosynthesis
Port		carry	transport, portable
Psych	Psycho	soul or spirit	psychiatrist, psyche, psychology
Qui	Quit	quiet or rest	acquittal, tranquility
Rupt		break	rupture, interrupt
Scope		see, inspect	telescope, microscopic
Scrib	Script	write	describe, transcription
Sens	Sent	feel	sensory, consent
Spect		look	spectate, circumspect
Struct		build	construct, obstruction
Techno	Tech	art or science	technical, technology
Tele		far	teleport, television
Therm		heat	thermometer, thermal
Vac		empty	vacation, evacuate
Vis	Vid	see	visual, video
Voc		speak or call	vocal, vocation

MEDICALLY SPECIFIC PREFIXES, ROOTS, AND SUFFIXES

We've covered a wide variety of prefixes, roots, and suffixes that you are likely familiar with even if you didn't realize it. That created a great foundation for delving into the medically specific prefixes, roots, and suffixes that you don't hear as frequently outside the scientific and medical community. Some of those below you have already seen, of course, but they are worth repeating.

Prefixes That Indicate Number or Size

Prefix	Meaning	Examples
Bi-	two	bicep, bisexual
Dipl/o-	two, double	diplopia, diplacusis
Hemi-	half	hemiacrosomia, hemialgia
Hyper-	over or more than usual	hyperthermia, hyperacidity
Hypo-	under or less than usual	hypothermia, hypoacusis
Iso-	equal, same	isodisomy, isoantigen
Macro-	large	macrocardius, macrocolon
Megal/o-	enlargement	megalgia, megalocephalic

(Continued)

Prefix	Meaning	Examples
Micro-	small	microabscess, microaneurysm
Mono-	one	monochromasia, monoarticular
Multi-	many	multienzyme, multicamerate
Nulli-	none	nullipara, nulligravida
Poly-	many	polyarthritis, polyalgesia
Semi-	half, partial	semipronation, semicoma
Tri-	three	triad, triacid
Uni-	one	unilateral, uniocular

Root Words That Indicate Color

Prefix	Meaning	Examples
Chlor/o-	green	chlorine
Cyan/o-	blue	cyanide
Erythr/o-	red	erythrean, erythrocyte
Leuk/o-	white	leukemia, leukosis
Melan/o-	black	melanemia
Xanth/o-	yellow	xanthemia

Prefixes That Indicate Direction or Location

Prefix	Meaning	Examples
Per-	through	perceptive
Peri-	around	periscope
Post-	behind, after	postmortem

(Continued)

Prefix	Meaning	Examples
Poster/o-	behind	posterior
Pre-	before, in front of	preanal, preaxial
Pro-	before	procelia
Retr/o-	behind, in back of	retrocolic, retrograde
Sub-	under	subabdominal, subcutaneous
Super-	beyond	supercilia, superficialis
Supra-	above	supraventricular, supraspinal
Syn-	together	synthetic, synactosis
Trans-	across	transbasal, transatrial
Ventr/o-	belly	ventricular, ventrolateral

Word Roots for Organs

Note: Some of the prefixes and suffixes covered in previous pages are used in the examples below.

Root	Meaning	Examples
Cardio	heart	electrocardiogram
Colo	large intestine	colitis, megacolon
Cysto	bladder	cystitis
Dento	teeth	dentist
Dermo	skin	dermatitis
Encephalo	brain	encephalitis
Entero	intestine	gastroenteritis
Gastro	stomach	gastritis

(Continued)

Medically Specific Prefixes, Roots, and Suffixes

Root	Meaning	Examples
Gingivo	gums	gingivitis
Glosso/Linguo	tongue	glossitis, lingual nerve
Hemo/Emia	blood	hematologist, anemia
Hepato	liver	hepatitis, hepatomegaly
Hystero/Metro	uterus	hysterectomy, endometritis
Masto/Mammo	breast	mammography, mastectomy
Nephro/Rene	kidney	nephrosis, renal artery
Oophoro	ovary	oophorectomy
Orchido	testis	orchiditis, orchidectomy
Osteo	bones	osteoporosis
Phlebo/Veno	veins	phlebitis, phlebotomy
Pneumo/Pulmo	lung	pneumonitis, pulmonologist
Procto	anus/rectum	proctitis, proctologist
Rhino	nose	rhinitis
Salpingo	uterine tubes	hysterosalpingogram
Stomato	mouth	stomatitis

ROOT WORDS AND AFFIXES IN ALPHABETICAL ORDER

What follows is a comprehensive list for quick reference. Many of these affixes show up in other sections of this book; if you hear or see a part of a word you can't recall, you can quickly look it up here.

A

Root/Affix	Meaning	Examples
A-, An-	not, without (alpha privative)	analgesic, apathy
Ab	from; away from	abduction
Abdomin-	of or relating to the abdomen	abdomen, abdominal
-ac	pertaining to; one afflicted with	cardiac, hydrophobiac
Acanth-	thorn or spine	acanthion, acanthocyte, acanthoma, acanthulus
Acou-	of or relating to hearing	Iacoumeter, acoustician, hyperacusis
Acr	extremity, topmost	acrocrany, acromegaly, acroosteolysis, acroposthia
-acusis	hearing	paracusis
-ad	toward, in the direction of	dorsad, ventrad

(Continued)

Root/Affix	Meaning	Examples
Ad-	at, increase, on, toward	adduction, addition
Aden	of or relating to a gland	adenocarcinoma, adenology, adenotome, adenotyphus
Adip	of or relating to fat or fatty tissue	adipocyte
Adren-	of or relating to the adrenal glands	adrenal artery
-aemia, -ema, Hemat	blood condition	anemia, hematology
Aer(o)	air, gas	aerosinusitis, aerodynamics
Aesthesi-	sensation	anesthesia, anesthesiologist
-al	pertaining to	abdominal, femoral
Alb	denoting a white or pale color	albino, tunica albica
Alge(si)-	pain	analgesic
-algia, Alg(i)o-	pain	lmyalgia
All-	denoting something as different or an addition	alloantigen, allopathy
Ambi-	denoting something involving both left and right side	ambidextrous
Amnio-	pertaining to the membranous fetal sac (amnion)	amniocentesis
Amph(i)	on both sides	amphicrania, amphismela, amphomycin
Amylo-	starchy, carbohydrate-related	amylase, amylophagia
An-	not, without (alpha privative)	analgesia
An-	anus	anal

Root/Affix	Meaning	Examples
Ana-	back, again, up	anaplasia
Andr	pertaining to a man	android, andrology, androgen
Angi	blood vessel	angiogram, angioplasty
Aniso-	describing something as unequal	anisocytosis, anisotropic
Ankyl-, Ancyl-	denoting something as crooked or bent	ankylosis
Ante-	describing something as positioned in front of another thing	antepartum
Anthropo-	human	anthropology
Anti-	describing something as against or opposed to another	antibody, antipsychotic
Apo-	away, separated from, derived from	apoptosis
Archi-	first, primitive	archinephron
Arsen(o)-	of or pertaining to a male; masculine	arsenoblast
Arteri(o)-	of or pertaining to an artery	arteriole, artery
Arthr-	of or pertaining to the joints, limbs	arthritis
Articul-	joint	articulation
-ary	pertaining to	biliary tract, coronary
-ase	enzyme	lactase
-asthenia	weakness	myasthenia gravis
Atel(o)-	imperfect or incomplete development	atelocardia

(Continued)

Root/Affix	Meaning	Examples
Ather-	fatty deposit, soft gruel-like deposit	atherosclerosis
-ation	process	medication, civilization
Atri-	an atrium (esp. heart atrium)	atrioventricular
Aur-	of or pertaining to the ear	aural
Aut-	self	autoimmune, autograph, autobiography, automatic
Aux(o)-	increase; growth	auxocardia: enlargement of the heart, auxology
Axill-	of or pertaining to the armpit (uncommon as a prefix)	axilla
Azo(to)-	nitrogenous compound	azothermia: raised temperature due to nitrogenous substances in blood

B

Root/Affix	Meaning	Examples
Bacilli-, Bacillus	rod-shaped	bacillus anthracis
Bacteri-	pertaining to bacteria	bacteriophage, bactericide
Balan-	of the glans penis or glans clitoridis	balanitis
Bas-	of or pertaining to base	basolateral
Bi-	twice, double	binary vision, bicycle, bisexual
Bio-	life	biology, biological
Blast-	germ or bud	blastomere
Blephar(o)-	of or pertaining to the eyelid	blepharoplasty
Brachi(o)-	of or relating to the arm	brachium of inferior colliculus
Brachy-	indicating "short" or less commonly "little"	brachycephalic
Brady-	"slow"	bradycardia
Bronch(i)-	of or relating to the bronchus	bronchitis, bronchiolitis obliterans
Bucc(o)-	of or pertaining to the cheek	buccolabial
Burs(o)-	bursa (fluid sac between the bones)	bursa, bursitis

C

Root/Affix	Meaning	Examples
Capill-	of or pertaining to hair	capillus
Capit-	pertaining to the head as a whole	capitation, decapitation
Carcin-	cancer	carcinoma
Cardi-	of or pertaining to the heart	cardiology
Carp-	of or pertaining to the wrist	carpopedal spasm, carpal, metacarpal
Cata-	down, under	cataract, catabolism, catacombs
-cele	pouching, hernia	hydrocele, varicocele
-centesis	surgical puncture for aspiration	amniocentesis
Cephal(o)-	of or pertaining to the head (as a whole)	cephalalgy, hydrocephalus
Cerat(o)-	of or pertaining to the cornu; a horn	ceratoid
Cerebell(o)-	of or pertaining to the cerebellum	cerebellum
Cerebr-	of or pertaining to the brain	cerebrology
Cervic-	of or pertaining to the neck or the cervix	cervicodorsal, cervical vertebrae
Cheil-	of or pertaining to the lips	angular cheilitis
Chem-	chemistry, drug	chemotherapy, chemistry, chemical
Chir-, Cheir-	of or pertaining to the hand	chiropractor
Chlor-	denoting a green color	chlorophyll

Root/Affix	Meaning	Examples
Chol(e)-	of or pertaining to bile	cholemia, cholecystitis
Cholecyst(o)-	of or pertaining to the gallbladder	cholecystectomy
Chondr(i)o-	cartilage, gristle, granule, granular	chondrocalcinosis
Chrom(ato)-	color	hemochromatosis
-cidal, -cide	killing, destroying	bacteriocidal, suicide, suicidal
Cili-	of or pertaining to the cilia, the eyelashes; eyelids	ciliary
Circum-	denoting something as 'around' another	circumcision
Cis-	on this side	cisgender
-clast	break	osteoclast
Clostr-	spindle	clostridium
Co-	with, together, in association	coenzymes, co-organization
-coccus	round, spherical	streptococcus
Col-, Colo-, Colono-	colon	colonoscopy
Colp(o)-	of or pertaining to the vagina	colposcopy
Com-	with, together	communicate
Contra-	against	contraindication
Cor-	with, together	corrective
Cor-	of or pertaining to the eye's pupil	corectomy

(Continued)

Root/Affix	Meaning	Examples
Cord(i)-	of or pertaining to the heart (uncommon as a prefix)	commotio cordis
Cornu-	applied to describing processes and parts of the body as likened or like horns	greater cornu
Coron(o)-	pertaining to the heart	coronary heart disease
Cortic(o)-	cortex, outer region	corticosteroid
Cost-	of or pertaining to the ribs	costochondral
Cox-	of or relating to hip, haunch, or hip joint	coxopodite
Crani(o)-	belonging or relating to the cranium	craniology
-crine, -crin(o)	to secrete	endocrine
Cry(o)-	cold	cryoablation, cryogenic
Cutane-	skin	subcutaneous
Cyan(o)-	having a blue color	cyanopsia
Cycl-	circle, cycle	cyclosis, cyclops, tricycle
Cyph(o)-	denotes something as bent (uncommon as a prefix)	cyphosis
Cyst(o)-, Cyst(i)-	of or pertaining to the urinary bladder	cystotomy
Cyt(o)-, -cyte	cell	cytokine, leukocyte, cytoplasm

D

Root/Affix	Meaning	Examples
Dacry(o)-	of or pertaining to tears	dacryoadenitis, dacryocystitis
-dactyl(o)-	of or pertaining to a finger, toe	dactylology, polydactyly
De-	from, down, or away from	dehydrate, demotion
Dent-	of or pertaining to teeth	dentist, dental
Dermat(o)-, Derm(o)-	of or pertaining to the skin	dermatology, epidermis, hypodermic, xeroderma
-desis	binding	arthrodesis
Dextr(o)-	right, on the right side	dextrocardia
Di-	two	diplopia,
Di-	apart, separation	dilation, distal, dilute
Dia-	through, during, across	dialysis
Dif-	apart, separation	different
Digit-	of or pertaining to the finger [rare as a root]	digit
Diplo-	twofold	diploid, diplosis
-dipsia	(condition of) thirst	dipsomania, hydroadipsia, oligodipsia, polydipsia
Dis-	separation, taking apart	dissection
Dors(o)-, Dors(i)-	of or pertaining to the back	dorsal, dorsocephalad
Dromo-	running, conduction, course	dromotropic, syndrome
Duodeno-	twelve	duodenal atresia, duodenum
Dura-	hard	dura mater

(Continued)

Root/Affix	Meaning	Examples
Dynam(o)-	force, energy, power	hand strength dynamometer, dynamics
-dynia	pain	vulvodynia
Dys-	bad, difficult, defective, abnormal	dysentery, dysphagia, dysphasia

E

Root/Affix	Meaning	Examples
-eal (see -al)	pertaining to	adenohypophyseal, corneal, esophageal, perineal
Ec-	out, away	ectopia, ectopic pregnancy
Ect(o)-	outer, outside	ectoblast, ectoderm, ectoplasm
-ectasia, -ectasis	expansion, dilation	bronchiectasis, telangiectasia
-ectomy	a surgical operation or removal of body part; resection, excision	mastectomy
-emesis	vomiting condition	hematemesis
-emia	blood condition	anemia
Encephal(o)-	of or pertaining to the brain; see also cerebra-	encephalogram
Endo-	denotes something as inside or within	endocrinology, endospore, endoskeleton
Eosin(o)-	having a red color	eosinophil granulocyte
Enter(o)-	of or pertaining to the intestine	gastroenterology
Epi-	on, upon	epicardium, epidermis, epidural, episclera, epistaxis, epidemic
Episi(o)-	of or pertaining to the pubic region, the loins	episiotomy
Erythr(o)-	having a red color	erythrocyte
-esophageal, Esophago-	gullet	esophagus
Esthesio-	sensation	esthesioneuroblastoma, esthesia

(Continued)

Root/Affix	Meaning	Examples
Eu-	true, good, well, new	eukaryote
Ex-	out of, away from	excision, except
Exo-	denotes being outside another	exophthalmos, exoskeleton, exoplanet
Extra-	outside	extradural hematoma, extraordinary, extreme

F

Root/Affix	Meaning	Examples
Faci-	of or pertaining to the face	facioplegic, facial
Fibr-	fiber	fibril, fibrin, fibrinous pericarditis, fibroblast, fibrosis
Fil-	fine, hair-like	filament, filum terminale
Foramen	Hole, opening, or aperture, particularly in bone	Foramen magnum
-form	Used to form adjectives indicating "having the form of"	Cruciform, cuneiform, falciform
Fore-	Before or ahead	Foregut, foreshadow
Fossa	a hollow or depressed area; a trench or channel	fossa ovalis
Front-	of or pertaining to the forehead	frontonasal

G

Root/Affix	Meaning	Examples
Galact-	milk	galactorrhea, galaxy
Gastr-	of or pertaining to the stomach	gastric bypass, gastroenterology
-gen	born in, from of a certain kind	heterogenous
-genic	formative; pertaining to producing	cardiogenic shock
Genu-	of or pertaining to the knee	genu valgum
-geusia	taste	ageusia, dysgeusia, hypergeusia, hypogeusia, parageusia
Gingiv-	of or pertaining to the gums	gingivitis
Glauc(o)-	having a grey or bluish-grey color	glaucoma
Gloss(o)-, Glott*o)-	of or pertaining to the tongue	glossology
Gluco-	sweet	glucocorticoid, glucose
Glyc-	sugar	glycolysis
Gnath-	of or pertaining to the jaw	gnathodynamometer
-gnosis	knowledge	diagnosis, prognosis
Gon-	seed, semen; reproductive	gonorrhea
-gram, -gramme	record or picture	angiogram, gramophone
-graph	instrument used to record data or picture	electrocardiograph, seismograph
-graphy	process of recording	angiography
Gyno-, Gynaeco-, Gyneco-	woman	gynecology, gynecomastia, gynoecium

H

Root/Affix	Meaning	Examples
Halluc-	to wander in mind	hallucinosis, hallucination
Hemat-, Haemato-, Haem-, Hem-	of or pertaining to blood	hematology, older form: haematology
Hema-, Hemo-	blood	hemal, hemoglobin
Hemangi-, Hemangio-	blood vessels	hemangioma
Hemi-	one-half	cerebral hemisphere
Hepat-, Hepatic-	of or pertaining to the liver	hepatology, hepatitis
Heter(o)-	denotes something as the other (of two), an addition, or different	heterogeneous
Hidr(o)-	sweat	hyperhidrosis
Hist(o)-, Histio-	tissue	histology
Home(o)-	similar	homeopathy
Hom(o)-	denotes something as "the same" as another or common	homosexuality, homozygote, homophobic
Humer(o)-	of or pertaining to the shoulder (or [rarely] the upper arm)	humerus
Hydr(o)-	water	hydrophobe, hydrogen
Hyper-	extreme or beyond normal	hypertension, hypertrichosis
Hyp(o)-	below normal	hypovolemia, hypoxia
Hyster(o)-	of or pertaining to the womb or the uterus	hysterectomy, hysteria

I

Root/Affix	Meaning	Examples
-iasis	condition, formation, or presence of	mydriasis
Iatr(o)-	of or pertaining to medicine or a physician (uncommon prefix but common as a suffix; see -iatry)	iatrochemistry, iatrogenesis
-iatry	denotes a field in medicine emphasizing a certain body component	podiatry, psychiatry
-ic	pertaining to	hepatic artery
-ics	organized knowledge, treatment	obstetrics
Idio-	self, one's own	idiopathic
Ileo-	ileum	ileocecal valve
Infra-	below	infrahyoid muscles
Inter-	between, among	interarticular ligament
Intra-	within	intramural
Ipsi-	same	ipsilateral
Irid(o)-	of or pertaining to the iris	iridectomy
Isch-	restriction	ischemia
Ischio-	of or pertaining to the ischium, the hip-joint	ischioanal fossa
-ism	condition, disease	dwarfism
-ismus	spasm, contraction	hemiballismus
Iso-	denoting something as being equal	isotonic

Root/Affix	Meaning	Examples
-ist	one who specializes in	pathologist
-ite	the nature of, resembling	dendrite
-itis	inflammation	tonsillitis
-ium	structure, tissue	pericardium

J & K

Root/Affix	Meaning	Examples
Juxta-, luxta-	near to, alongside, or next to	juxtaglomerular apparatus
Kal-	potassium	hyperkalemia
Kary-	nucleus	eukaryote
Kerat-	cornea (eye or skin)	keratoscope
Kine-	movement	akinetopsia, kinesthesia
Koil-	hollow	koilocyte
Kyph-	humped	kyphoscoliosis

L

Root/Affix	Meaning	Examples
Labi-	of or pertaining to the lip	labiodental
Lacrim(o)-	tear	lacrimal canaliculi
Lact(i)-, Lact(o)-	milk	lactation
Lapar(o)-	of or pertaining to the abdominal wall, flank	laparotomy
Laryng(o)-	of or pertaining to the larynx, lower throat cavity with the voice box	larynx
Latero-	lateral	lateral pectoral nerve
Lei(o)-	smooth	leiomyoma
-lepsis, -lepsy	attack, seizure	epilepsy, narcolepsy
Lept(o)-	light, slender	leptomeningeal
Leuc(o)-, Leuk(o)-	denoting a white color	leukocyte
Lingu(a)-, Lingu(o)-	of or pertaining to the tongue	linguistics
Lip(o)-	fat	liposuction
Liss(os)-	smooth	lissencephaly
Lith(o)-	stone, calculus	lithotripsy
Log(o)-	speech	dialog, catalog, logos
-logist	denotes someone who studies a certain field (the field of -logy); a specialist; one who treats	oncologist, pathologist
-logy	denotes academic study or practice of a certain field	hematology, urology

(Continued)

Root/Affix	Meaning	Examples
Lumb(o)-, Lumb(a)-	of or relating to the part of the trunk between the lowest ribs and the pelvis.	lumbar vertebrae
Lymph(o)-	lymph	lymphedema
Lys(o)-, -lytic	dissolution	lysosome
-lysis	destruction, separation	paralysis

M

Root/Affix	Meaning	Examples
Macr(o)-	large, long	macrophage
-malacia	softening	osteomalacia
Mamm(o)-	of or pertaining to the breast	mammogram
Mammill(o)-	of or pertaining to the nipple	mammillaplasty, mammillitis
Manu-	of or pertaining to the hand	manufacture
Mast(o)-	of or pertaining to the breast	mastectomy
Meg(a)-, Megal(o)-, -megaly	enlargement, million	splenomegaly, megameter
Melan(o)-	having a black color	melanin
Melos	extremity, limb	erythromelalgia
Mening(o)-	membrane	meningitis
Men-	month, menstrual cycle	menopause, menorrhagia
Mer-	part	merocrine, meroblastic
Mes-	middle	medoderm
Met, Meta-	after, besides, beyond, change	metacarpal, metacarpus, metacromion, metanephros
-meter	instrument used to measure or count	sphygmoma nometer, thermometer
-metry	process of measuring, meter + y (see -meter)	optometry
Metr-	pertaining to conditions or instruments of the uterus	metrorrhagia
Micr-	millionth; denoting something as small, relating to smallness	microscope

(Continued)

Root/Affix	Meaning	Examples
Milli-	thousandth	milliliter
Mon-	single	infectious mononucleosis
Morph-	form, shape	morphology
Muscul(o)-	muscle	musculoskeletal system
My(o)-	of or relating to muscle	myoblast
Myc(o)-	fungus	onychomycosis
Myel(o)-	of or relating to bone marrow or the spinal cord	myelin sheath, myeloblast
Myl(o)-	of or relating to molar teeth or the lower jaw	mylohyoid nerve
Myri-	ten thousand	myriad
Myring(o)-	eardrum	myringotomy
Myx(o)-	mucus	myxoma

N

Root/Affix	Meaning	Examples
Nan(o)-	dwarf, small	nanogram, nanosecond
Narc(o)-	numb, sleep	narcolepsy
Nas(o)-	of or pertaining to the nose	nasal
Nat(o)-	birth	neonatology
Necr(o)	death	necrosis, necrotizing fasciitis
Neo-	new	neoplasm
Nephr(o)-	of or pertaining to the kidneys	nephrology
Nerv-	of or pertaining to nerves and the nervous system (uncommon as a root: neuro- mostly always used)	nerve, nervous system
Neur(i)-, Neur(o)-	of or pertaining to nerves and the nervous system	neurofibromatosis
Noci-	pain, injury, hurt	nociception
Normo-	normal	normocapnia

O

Root/Affix	Meaning	Examples
Ocul(o)-	of or pertaining to the eye	oculist
Odont(o)-	of or pertaining to teeth	orthodontist
Odyn(o)-	pain	stomatodynia
-oesophageal, Oesophago-	gullet	oesophagus
-oid	resemblance to	sarcoidosis
-ole	small or little	arteriole
Olig(o)-	having little, having few	oligotrophy
Om(o)-	shoulder	omoplate
-oma (singular), -omata (plural)	tumor, mass, fluid collection	sarcoma, teratoma, mesothelioma
Omphal(o)-	of or pertaining to the navel, the umbilicus	omphalotomy
Onco-	tumor, bulk, volume	oncology
Onych(o)-	of or pertaining to the nail (of a finger or toe)	onychophagy
Oo-	of or pertaining to a women's egg, the ovum	oogenesis
Oophor(o)-	of or pertaining to the woman's ovary	oophorectomy
Ophthalm(o)-	of or pertaining to the eye	ophthalmology
Opistho-	back, behind, rear	opisthotonus
-opsy	examination or inspection	biopsy, autopsy

Root/Affix	Meaning	Examples
Optic(o)-	of or relating to chemical properties of the eye	opticochemical, biopsy
Or(o)-	of or pertaining to the mouth	oral
-or	person, agent	doctor
Orchi(o)-, Orchid(o)-, Orch(o)-	testis	orchiectomy, orchidectomy
Orth(o)-	denoting something as straight or correct	orthodontist
-osis	a condition, disease, or increase	harlequin-type ichthyosis, psychosis, osteoporosis
Ossi-, Osse-	bone, bony	peripheral ossifying fibroma, osseous
Ost(e)-, Oste(o)-	bone	osteoporosis, osteoarthritis
Ot(o)-	of or pertaining to the ear	otology
-ous	pertaining to	porous
Ovari(o)-	of or pertaining to the ovaries	ovariectomy
Ovo-, Ovi-, Ov-	of or pertaining to the eggs, the ovum	ovogenesis
Oxo-	addition of oxygen	oxobutanoic acid
Oxy-	sharp, acid, acute, oxygen	oxygenated, oxvcodone

P

Root/Affix	Meaning	Examples
Pachy-	thick	pachyderma
Palpebr-	of or pertaining to the eyelid (uncommon as a root)	palpebra
Pan-, Pant(o)-	denoting something as complete or containing everything; all	panophobia, panopticon, pancytopenia (deficiency in all blood cell types: erythrocytes, leukocytes, thrombocytes)
Papill-	of or pertaining to the nipple (of the chest/breast)	papillitis
Papul(o)-	indicating papulosity, a small elevation or swelling in the skin, a pimple, swelling	papulation
Para-	alongside of	paracyesis
-paresis	slight paralysis	hemiparesis
Parvo-	small	parvovirus
Path(o)-	disease	pathology
-pathy	denoting (with a negative sense) a disease or disorder	sociopathy, neuropathy
Pauci-	few	pauci-immune
Pector-	breast or chest	pectoralgia, pectoriloquy, pectorophony
Ped-, Ped, -pes	of or pertaining to the foot; footed	pedoscope
Ped-, Pedo-	of or pertaining to the child	pediatrics. pedophilia
Pelv(i)-, Pelv(o)-	hip bone	pelvis
-penia	deficiency	osteopenia

Root/Affix	Meaning	Examples
Peo-	of or pertaining to the penis	peotomy
-pepsia	denoting something relating to digestion, or the digestive tract.	dyspepsia
Per-	through	percutaneous
Peri-	denoting something with a position, surrounding or being around another	
-phagia, -phage	denoting conditions relating to eating or ingestion	sarcophagia
Phago-	eating, devouring	phagocyte
Phagist-	denoting a person who feeds on the first element or part of the word	lotophagi
-phagy	Denoting feeding on, the first element or part of the word	hematophagy
Phall-	phallus, penis	aphallia
Pharmac-	drug, medication	pharmacology
Pharyng-	of or pertaining to the (blood) veins, a vein	phlebography, phlebotomy
-phil(ia)	attraction for	hemophilia
Phleb-	of or pertaining to the (blood) veins, a vein	phlebography, phlebotomy
-phobia	exaggerated fear, sensitivity, aversion	arachnophobia
Phon-	sound	phonograph, symphony

(Continued)

Root/Affix	Meaning	Examples
Phos-	of or pertaining to light or its chemical properties, now historic and used rarely. see the common root phot- below.	phosphene
Phot-	of or pertaining to light	photopathy
Phren-, Phrenic-	the mind	phrenic nerve, schizophrenia
Phyllo-	leaf-like	phyllodes tumor, phyllotaxis
-phyte, Phyto-	to grow	hydrophyte
Pia	soft	pia mater
Piri-	pear	piriformis muscle
-plasia	formation, development	achondroplasia
-plasty	surgical repair, reconstruction	rhinoplasty
-plegia	paralysis	paraplegia
Pleio-	More, excessive, multiple	pleiomorphism
Pleur-	of or pertaining to the ribs	pleurogenous
-plexy	stroke or seizure	cataplexy
Pne-, Pneum-	air, breath, lung	apnea, pneumatology, pneumonocyte, pneumonia
Pod-, -pod, -pus	of or pertaining to the foot, footed	podiatry
-poiesis	production	hematopoiesis
Polio-	having a grey color	poliomyelitis
Poly-	denoting a plurality of something	polymyositis
Por-	pore, porous	pore

Root/Affix	Meaning	Examples
Porphyr-	denoting a purple color	porphyroblast
Post-	denoting something as after or behind another	postoperation, postmortem
Pre-	denotes something as before another	premature birth (in [physical] position or time)
Presby-	old age	presbyopia, presbycusis
Prim-	denoting something as first or most important	primary
Pro-	denoting something as before another (in [physical] position or time)	procephalic
Proct-	anus, rectum	proctology
Prosop-	face	prosopagnosia
Prot-	denoting something as first or most important	protoneuron
Pseud-	denoting something false or fake	pseudoephedrine
Psor-	itching	psoriasis
Psych-	of or pertaining to the mind	psychology, psychiatry
Ptero-, Ptery-	pertaining to a wing; wing-shaped	lateral pterygoid plate
-ptosis	falling, drooping, downward placement, prolapse	apoptosis, nephroptosis
Ptyal-, Ptyalo-	saliva, salivary glands, sialaden	ptyalolithiasis
-ptysis	spitting	hemoptysis, the spitting of blood derived from the lungs or bronchial tubes
Pulmon-, Pulmo-	of or relating to the lungs	pulmonary

(Continued)

Root/Affix	Meaning	Examples
Py-	pus	pyometra
Pyel-	pelvis	pyelonephritis
Pykno-	thicken (as the nucleus does in early stages of cell death)	pyknosis
Pylor-	gate	pyloric sphincters
Pyr-	fever	antipyretic

Q & R

Root/Affix	Meaning	Examples
Quadr(i)	four	quadriceps
Radi	radiation	radiowave
Radic-	referring to the beginning or the root, of a structure, usually a nerve or a vein	radiculopathy
Re	again, back	relapse
Rect	rectum	rectal, rectum
Ren	of or pertaining to the kidney	renal
Reticul(o)	net	reticulocyte
Retro	backward, behind	retroversion, retroverted
Rhabd(o)	rod shaped, striated	rhabdomyolysis
Rhachi(o)-	spine	rachial, rachialgia, rachidian, rachiopathy
Rhin(o)-	of or pertaining to the nose	rhinoceros, rhinoplasty
Rhod(o)	denoting a rose-red color	rhodophyte
-rrhage, -rrhagia	burst forth, rapid flow (of blood, usually)	hemorrhage, menorrhagia
-rrhaphy	surgical suturing	hymenorrhaphy, neurorrhaphy
-rrhea	flowing, discharge	galactorrhea, diarrhea
-rrhexis	rupture	karyorrhexis
-rrhoea	flowing, discharge	diarrhoea (UK), diarrhea (US)
Rubr(o)-	of or pertaining to the red nucleus of the brain	rubrospinal
-rupt	break or burst	erupt, interrupt

S

Root/Affix	Meaning	Examples
Salping(o)-	of or pertaining to tubes (e.g., fallopian tubes)	salpingectomy, salpingopharyngeus muscle
Sangui-, Sanguine-	of or pertaining to blood	sanguine
Sapro-	relating to putrefaction or decay.	saprogenic
Sarco-	muscular, flesh-like	sarcoma, sarcoidosis
Schist(o)-	split, cleft	schistocyte
Schiz(o)-	denoting something split or double-sided	schizophrenia
Scler(o)-	hard	scleroderma
-sclerosis	hardening	atherosclerosis, multiple sclerosis
Scoli(o)-	twisted	scoliosis
-scope	instrument for viewing	stethoscope
-scopy	process of viewing	endoscopy
Scoto-	darkness	scotopic, vision
Semi-	one-half, partly	semiconscious
Sial(o)-	saliva, salivary gland	sialagogue
Sigmoid(o)-	sigmoid, s-shaped curvature	sigmoid colon
Sinistr(o)-	left, left side	sinistrodextral
Sinus-	of or pertaining to the sinus	sinusitis
Sito-	food, grain	sitophobia
Somat(o)-, Somatico-	body, bodily	somatic

Root/Affix	Meaning	Examples
Somn(o)	sleep	insomniac
-spadias	slit, fissure	hypospadias, epispadias
Spasmo-	spasm	spasmodic dysphonia
Sperma-, Spermo-, Spermato-	semen, spermatozoa	spermatogenesis
Splanchn(i)-, splanchn(o)-	viscera	splanchnology
Splen(o)-	spleen	splenectomy
Spondyl(o)-	of or pertaining to the spine, the vertebra	spondylitis
Squamos(o)-	denoting something as full of scales or scaly	squamous cell
-stalsis	contraction	peristalsis
-stasis	stopping, standing	cytostasis, homeostasis
-staxis	dripping, trickling	angilostaxis
Sten(o)-	denoting something as narrow in shape; pertaining to narrowness	stenography
-stenosis	abnormal narrowing of a blood vessel or other tubular organ or structure	restenosis, stenosis
Steth-	of or pertaining to the upper chest, the area above the breast and under the neck	stethoscope
Stom-, Stomat-	of or pertaining to the mouth; an artificially created opening	stomatogastric, stomatognathic system
-stomy	creation of an opening	colostomy

(Continued)

Root/Affix	Meaning	Examples
Sub-	beneath, under	subcutaneous tissue
Super-	in excess, above, superior	superior vena cava
Supra-	above, excessive	supraorbital vein
Sy-, Syl-, Sym-, Syn-, Sys-	indicating similarity, likeness, or being together; assimilates before some consonants (e.g., before i to Syl-, s to Sys-, before a labial consonant to Sym-)	symptom, synalgia, synesthesia, syssarcosis

T

Root/Affix	Meaning	Examples
Tachy-	denoting something as fast, irregularly fast	tachycardia
-tension, -tensive	pressure	hypertension
Terato-	monster	teratoma, teratogen
Tetan-	rigid, tense	tetanus
Thec-	case, sheath	intrathecal
Thel-	of or pertaining to a nipple (uncommon as a prefix)	theleplasty, thelarche
Thely-	denoting something as relating to a woman, feminine	thelygenous
Therap-	treatment	hydrotherapy, therapeutic
Therm(o)-	heat	hypothermia
Thorac(i)-, Thorac(o)-, Thoracico-	of or pertaining to the upper chest, chest; the area above the breast and under the neck	thoracic, thorax
Thromb(o)-	of or relating to a blood clot, clotting of blood	thrombus, thrombocytopenia
Thyr(o)-	thyroid	thyrotropin
Thym-	emotions	dysthymia
-tic	pertaining to	acoustic
Toco-	childbirth	tocolytic
-tomy	act of cutting; incising, incision	gastrotomy
Ton-	tone, tension, pressure	tonus
Top(o)-	place, topical	topical anesthetic

(Continued)

Root/Affix	Meaning	Examples
Tort(i)-	twisted	torticollis
Tox(i)-, Tox(o)-, Toxic(o)-	toxin, poison	toxoplasmosis
Trache(a)-	trachea	tracheotomy
Trachel(o)-	of or pertaining to the neck	tracheloplasty
Trans-	denoting something as moving or situated across or through	transfusion
Tri-	three	triangle, triceps
Trich(i)-, Trichia, Trich(o)-	of or pertaining to hair, hair-like structure	trichocyst
-tripsy	crushing	lithotripsy
-trophy	nourishment, development	pseudohypertrophy
-tropic	turned toward, with an orientation toward, having an affinity for, affecting	phototropic (taking a particular direction under the influence of light)
Tympan(o)-	eardrum	tympanocentesis

U & V

Root/Affix	Meaning	Examples
-ula, -ule	small	nodule
Ultra	beyond, excessive	ultrasound, ultraviolet
Umbilic-	of or pertaining to the navel, the umbilicus	umbilical
Ungui	of or pertaining to the nail, a claw	unguiform, ungual
Un(i)	one	unilateral hearing loss
Ur-	of or pertaining to urine, the urinary system	antidiuretic, diuresis, diuretic, dysuria, enuresis, polyurea, polyuria, uraemia/uremia, uremic, ureter, urethra, urology
Urin-	of or pertaining to urine, the urinary system	uriniferous
Uter(o)-	of or pertaining to the uterus or womb	uterus
Vagin	of or pertaining to the vagina	vaginal epithelium
Varic(o)	swollen or twisted vein	varicose
Vas(o)	duct, blood vessel	vasoconstriction
Vasculo	blood vessel	vasculopathy
Ven-	of or pertaining to the veins, venous blood, and the vascular system	venule, venospasm
Ventr(o)-	of or pertaining to the belly, the stomach cavities	ventrodorsal
Ventricul(o)-	of or pertaining to the ventricles; any hollow region inside an organ	cardiac ventriculography, atrioventricular node
-version	turning	anteversion, retroversion

(Continued)

Root/Affix	Meaning	Examples
Vesic(o)	of or pertaining to the bladder	vesical arteries
Viscer(o)-	of or pertaining to the internal organs, the viscera	viscera

X, Y, & Z

Root/Affix	Meaning	Examples
Xanth(o)-	having a yellow color, especially an abnormally yellow color	xanthopathy
Xen(o)-	foreign, different	xenograft
Xer(o)-	dry, desert-like	xerostomia, xeroderma
Xiph-	sword	xiphisternum, xiphoid, xiphoidalgia
-y	condition or process of	surgery
Ze-	boil	eczema
Zo(o)-	animal, animal life	zoology
Zym(o)-	fermentation	enzyme, lysozyme

ANATOMICAL POSITIONS

We've covered the anatomy of words themselves and how to dissect and decipher the prefixes, roots, and suffixes. Now, we'll dive into the anatomy of the human body, how the terminology is used, and what it specifically means in a medical setting.

The anatomy of the human body and the discrete structures within it are described in part by their spatial orientations and relationships. Accordingly, the terms used to describe the relative positions of anatomical structures to one another are also used to describe specific regions of individual anatomical structures. In the definitions of these terms, some overlap exists, and occasionally, they may be used interchangeably. Most of the terms are best understood as pairs of opposing directions or relative locations. Below, we've broken down some of the most common pairs.

Dorsal vs. Ventral: "Dorsal" means toward the back of the body, and "ventral" means toward the front of the body. At the outer body surface, the back of the head, neck, torso, upper and lower legs and arms, the back of the hands and the upper surface and the top (vs. the soles) of the feet are the dorsal exterior surfaces. The most significant dorsal region landmarks are the midline of the spine and the shoulder blades, or left and right scapulae.

The exterior ventral surfaces are the front of the neck, chest, abdomen, pelvis, upper and lower arms and upper and lower legs, and the soles of the feet. Prominent ventral surfaces landmarks include the trachea (or windpipe) in the midline ventral neck, the sternum (or breastbone), the clavicles (or collarbones), the breasts in the ventral thorax (chest), the umbilicus (belly button) in the midline of the ventral abdomen, and the external genitalia in the ventral pelvis. The ventral surfaces of the arms are the surfaces that face upward when the arms are extended straight out with the palms facing upward.

Important dorsal/ventral regions are the dorsal and ventral regions of the spine and spinal cord, and the dorsum of the hands and feet (vs. the palms of the hands and the soles of the feet).

Anterior vs. Posterior: These terms are largely analogous to the terms dorsal and ventral, but are usually the terms preferentially used to describe relative positions. Commonly, one structure is defined as being "anterior to" or "posterior to" another structure rather than saying "dorsal to" or "ventral to." For instance, the esophagus is correctly described as being located "dorsal to" the heart, but the esophagus is usually described as located "posterior to" the heart, and conversely, the heart is located "anterior to" the esophagus.

Notable anatomical regions identified with these terms include the anterior and posterior pituitary (sub regions of the pituitary gland) and the coronary arteries (arteries that supply oxygenated blood to the muscle tissue of the heart); the left anterior descending coronary artery is one example.

Lateral vs. Medial: "Lateral" means to the side or the side(s) of. "Medial" means toward the center or closer to the midline. Lateral and medial are often used in combination other positional terms to produce a more precisely defined location (e.g., dorsolateral, ventromedial, anterolateral, etc.) The ventromedial hypothalamus is a notable region described in this manner.

One anatomical structure is commonly said to be located lateral or medial to another anatomical structure. Externally, the major lateral regions are the lateral chest regions, the lateral abdominal regions, and the lateral thigh and knee regions. The prominent medial regions of the external surfaces of the body are the medial thigh and medial knee regions.

Inferior vs. Superior: "Superior" means above, over, or toward the top of the head. "Inferior" means below, underneath, or toward the feet. These terms can be combined with other positional terms to identify more precise and discrete anatomical regions, such as the anterior superior ischial spine region of the pelvis.

Rostral vs. Caudal: This pair of descriptive terms is somewhat analogous to the terms superior and inferior. "Rostral" means toward the head or cranium, and "Caudal" means toward the pelvis or the base of the spine. These terms are rarely used comparatively. Instead, the terms are most often used in reference to the regions between the head and pelvis, and are not used to describe the appendages (arms and legs).

Superficial vs. Deep: "Superficial" means shallow, or toward the surface of, or closer to the skin. "Deep" means closer to the center of or farther from the surface of. Superficial body structures include skin, hair, facial structures (e.g., eyes, nose, and mouth), nipples of the breast, the umbilicus, and external genitalia.

The deepest structures in the appendages of the body (arms and legs) include the medullary cavities of the long bones. The deepest regions of the skull are the ventricles at the center of the brain. With respect to the external body surfaces, the heart, digestive organs, kidneys, urinary bladder, and female reproductive organs are deep structures.

When describing relative positions of two or more anatomical structures or locations, the superficial structure or location is closer to the external surface of the body compared to the deep structure or location. For example, the esophagus is posterior to the trachea, but describing the esophagus as being "deep to the trachea" is equally correct.

Proximal vs. Distal: "Proximal" means close or nearer to, and "distal" means distant, farther away from, or toward the end of. The reference point used to define proximal or distal varies depending on what is being described. In the broadest sense, proximal is closer to the center mass of the body within the deep chest or abdomen, while distal is nearer to the tips of the toes or fingers, or the top of the head.

Usually, the reference point is more specific. The aorta, the main artery of the body, for instance, begins at the heart and passes from the chest into the abdomen with a first major branch at the femoral arteries. In this case, the reference point is the heart; the abdominal aorta is proximal to the femoral arteries and distal to the thoracic aorta with respect to proximity to the heart. In the kidneys, small filtering units have structures called renal tubules. The tubule is divided into proximal and distal renal tubule segments. In this case, the reference point is Bowman's capsule, a central region of these small filtering units of the kidney.

Prone vs. Supine: This term pair defines two general positions of the entire human body. The "supine" position occurs when lying flat on one's back, arms and legs are extended (straight, not bent at a joint such as the knee or elbow). The palms of the hands are facing upward, and the heels of the feet are in contact with the ground.

The "prone" position is the reverse of the supine position, occurring when one is lying flat and face down, with the palms of the hands and the tops of the feet in contact with the ground. In the supine position all the ventral anatomical surfaces of the body are facing upward. For the prone position, the reverse is true: all the dorsal surfaces of the body are facing upward (except for the upper arms, where the lateral surfaces face upward).

CROSS SECTIONS OF THE BODY

The anatomy of the body can be visually displayed as cross sections, either of the entire body or of body structures (e.g., heart or brain). These sections are defined in relation to a human body being in an upright standing position. Three primary types of cross-sectional views exist: the transverse, the sagittal, and the coronal cross-sectional views. Below, the image depicts all three planes.

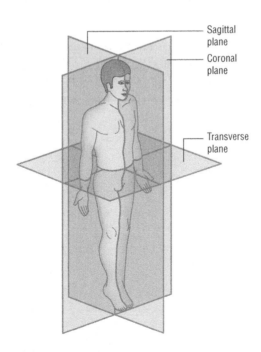

Sagittal
plane

Coronal
plane

Transverse
plane

Transverse sections are the views represented as if the body has been sliced cleanly in two on the horizontal plane. A mid-sagittal view will divide the upper body (head, arms, chest, and upper abdomen) and the lower body (lower abdomen, pelvis, and legs) at about the waistline of a typical individual. Cross-sections of the body may occur at any higher or lower horizontal height, moving either toward the top of the head or toward the soles of the feet.

Sagittal sections divide the body into a left and a right side. The mid-sagittal section will divide the body into equal right and left sides, as if a knife had cut cleanly through the body beginning at the top of the head and then proceeded downward through the midline axis of the body. The left section will include the left side of the face, neck, chest, abdomen, and pelvis, and the left leg. The reverse is true for the right section of the body.

Coronal sections are identical to sagittal sections except that the dissection plane is rotated by 90 degrees. This rotation results in a transection of the body that results in a front, ventral, or anterior section and a back, dorsal, or posterior section. A mid-coronal section divides the body into front and back sections at the midline of the body.

Any sagittal section of the body may be obtained by moving the dissection plane parallel and lateral to the mid-sagittal section. Any coronal section of the body may be obtained by moving the dissection plane parallel and lateral to the mid-coronal section.

ANATOMICAL DIRECTION AND MOTION

Nearly all voluntary movements of the human body occur through muscle contractions that result in motions of bones at joints designed for body movement (notable exceptions are facial expression movements and the motion of the diaphragm during breathing).

Generally, these motions refer to movement of the arms and legs (the appendages), but considerable numbers and types of movements occur along the skull-spine and spine-pelvis axis. The appendages are capable of complex motions, particularly at the shoulder, wrist, and ankle regions.

Flexion vs. Extension: At a joint, the adjacent ends of bones can move in ways that cause the joint angle between the bones to increase (open) or decrease (close) in a simple hinge-like fashion, usually within a maximum range of 180 degrees. The simple, hinge-like joint motion notably occurs at the elbow and knee joints, but most joints can produce this motion.

Extension is the increase in the angle of the joint (opening or extending out). Flexion is the opposite or reverse of extension. Flexion at a joint causes the bones at the joint to move in a manner that causes the joint angle to decrease (close or bend inward). Below, the image depicts flexion and extension movements at various parts of the body.

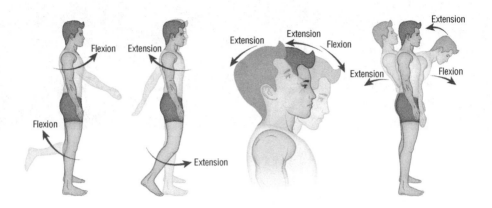

Abduction vs. Adduction: This type of motion is almost always in reference to motion of the upper arms at the shoulder joints and the upper legs at the hip joints. Abduction results in movement of the arms or legs outward, away from the midlines of the body. Adduction, the reverse of the motion of abduction, involves the movement of arms or legs toward the midlines of the body. Below, the image depicts these motions at the shoulder joint.

Medial Rotation vs. Lateral Rotation: "Lateral" means away from the midline, and "medial" means toward the midline. Any rotation toward the midline is a medial rotation, and any rotation away from the midline is a lateral rotation. Below, the image depicts these motions.

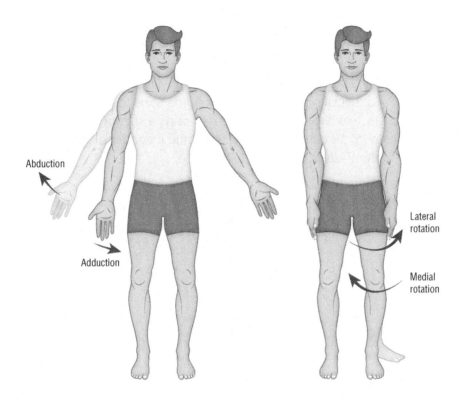

Dorsiflexion vs. Plantar Flexion: These movements involve the entire foot in relation to the ankle. "Dorsiflexion" means flexing the foot upward or superiorly. Conversely, "plantar flexion" means pointing the foot downward or inferiorly. Below, the image depicts these motions.

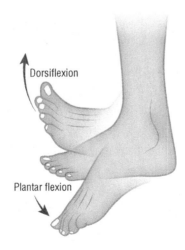

Pronation vs. Supination: In plain English terms, "prone" means being face down, and supine means being face up. When related to the hand, pronation simply means palm down and supination means palm up. Easy enough, right? But the identifying pronation and supination of the ankle can cause confusion with lateral and medial rotations. Pronation of the ankle to foot means a shift "inward" occurs, and supination of the ankle means a shift or angle where the weight is shifted to the outside the ankle. Below, the image depicts pronation and supination of the ankle on the RIGHT foot.

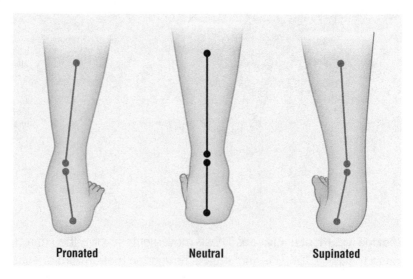

Pronated   Neutral   Supinated

REGIONS OF THE BODY

(Note: All regions in the lists are in order of superior to inferior.)

Head Regions

The cranial region encompasses the upper part of the head, while the facial region encompasses the lower half of the head, beginning below the ears.

- **Cephalic region:** the entire head region
- **Occipital region:** back of the head
- **Frontal region:** forehead
- **Orbital or ocular region:** eyes
- **Buccal region:** cheeks
- **Auricle or otic region:** ears
- **Nasal region:** nose
- **Oral region:** mouth
- **Mental region:** chin
- **Cervical region:** neck

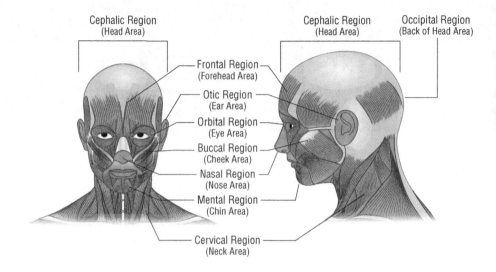

Cephalic Region
(Head Area)

Cephalic Region
(Head Area)

Occipital Region
(Back of Head Area)

Frontal Region
(Forehead Area)

Otic Region
(Ear Area)

Orbital Region
(Eye Area)

Buccal Region
(Cheek Area)

Nasal Region
(Nose Area)

Mental Region
(Chin Area)

Cervical Region
(Neck Area)

Trunk Regions

- **Thoracic region:** the chest
- **Mammary region:** each breast
- **Sternal region:** the sternum
- **Abdominal region:** the stomach area
- **Umbilicus, or naval**, is located at the center of the abdomen.
- **Coxal region:** the belt line
- **Pubic region:** the area above the genitals
- **Cervical region:** the neck
- **Scapular region:** the scapulae and the area around
- **Dorsal region:** the upper back
- **Lumbar region:** the lower back
- **Sacral region:** the end of the spine, directly above the buttocks
- **Acromial region:** the shoulder
- **Brachial region:** the upper arm
- **Olecranal region:** the back of the elbow
- **Antebrachial region:** the back of the arm
- **Manual or manus region:** the back of the hand

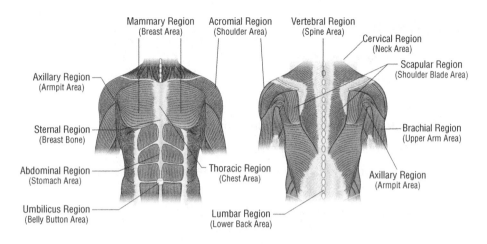

Mammary Region
(Breast Area)

Acromial Region
(Shoulder Area)

Vertebral Region
(Spine Area)

Cervical Region
(Neck Area)

Scapular Region
(Shoulder Blade Area)

Axillary Region
(Armpit Area)

Sternal Region
(Breast Bone)

Brachial Region
(Upper Arm Area)

Abdominal Region
(Stomach Area)

Thoracic Region
(Chest Area)

Axillary Region
(Armpit Area)

Umbilicus Region
(Belly Button Area)

Lumbar Region
(Lower Back Area)

Pelvic and Leg Regions

- **Inguinal or groin region:** between the legs and the genitals
- **Pubic region:** the genitals and surrounding areas
- **Gluteal region:** the buttocks
- **Gemoral region:** the thigh
- **Popliteal region:** the back of the knee
- **Sural region:** the back of the lower leg
- **Lumbar region:** the lower back, vertebrae L1 through L5
- **Sacral region:** the portion of spine between lower back and tailbone
- **Coxal region:** the lateral side of hips

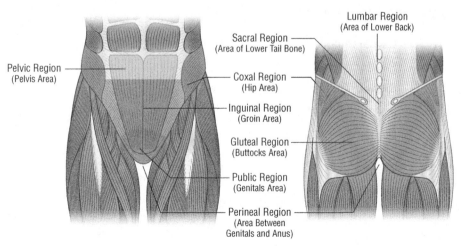

Lumbar Region
(Area of Lower Back)

Sacral Region
(Area of Lower Tail Bone)

Pelvic Region
(Pelvis Area)

Coxal Region
(Hip Area)

Inguinal Region
(Groin Area)

Gluteal Region
(Buttocks Area)

Public Region
(Genitals Area)

Perineal Region
(Area Between
Genitals and Anus)

Upper Limb Regions

- **Axillary region:** the armpit
- **Brachial region:** the upper arm
- **Antecubital region:** the front of the elbow
- **Antebrachial region:** the forearm
- **Acromial region:** the shoulder
- **Scapular region:** the upper thoracic region on the dorsal surface of the rib cage
- **Olecranal region:** the back of the elbow

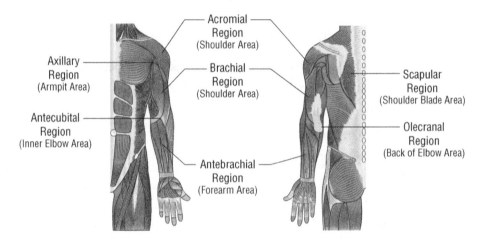

Hand and Wrist Regions

- **Carpal region:** the wrist
- **Palmar region:** the palm
- **Digital/phalangeal region:** the fingers
- **Pollex region:** the thumb
- **Manus region:** the hand area

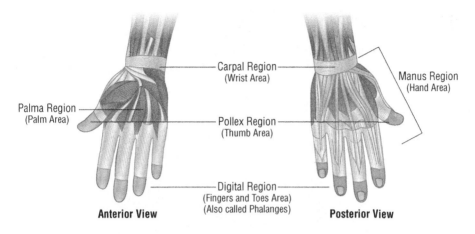

Carpal Region
(Wrist Area)

Manus Region
(Hand Area)

Palma Region
(Palm Area)

Pollex Region
(Thumb Area)

Digital Region
(Fingers and Toes Area)
(Also called Phalanges)

Anterior View

Posterior View

Leg Regions

- **Femoral region:** the thighs
- **Patellar region:** the knee
- **Crural region:** the shin area of the leg
- **Fibular region:** the outside of the lower leg
- **Gluteal region:** the buttocks
- **Popliteal region:** the back of the knee
- **Sural region:** the back of the lower leg

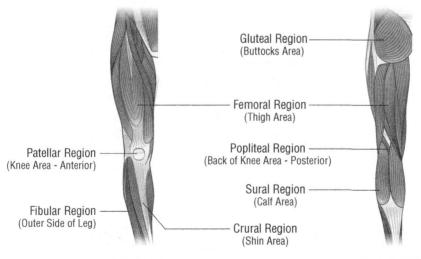

Gluteal Region
(Buttocks Area)

Femoral Region
(Thigh Area)

Patellar Region
(Knee Area - Anterior)

Popliteal Region
(Back of Knee Area - Posterior)

Sural Region
(Calf Area)

Fibular Region
(Outer Side of Leg)

Crural Region
(Shin Area)

Anterior View

Posterior View

Abdominal Regions

Specific to the abdominal area, sub-regions exist within this area. This important area of the body includes additional details due to the internal organs in and around the abdomen.

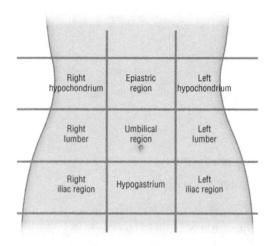

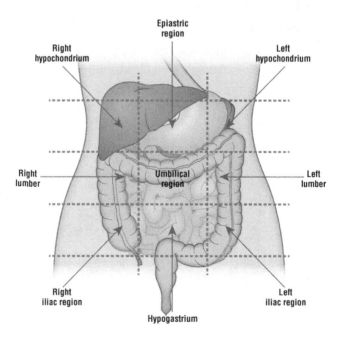

Feet and Ankle Regions

- **Tarsal region:** the ankle
- **Pedal region:** the foot
- **Digital/phalangeal region:** the toes
- **Hallux:** the "big" toe
- **Calcaneal region:** the heel
- **Plantar region:** the sole of the foot

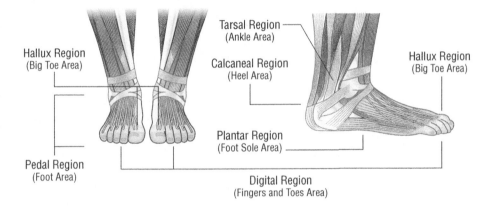

CAVITIES
OF THE BODY

Two major cavities exist in the human body: the **dorsal** and the **ventral** body cavities.

The Dorsal Cavity

The dorsal cavity is a body cavity located on the posterior (back) side of the human body. The ventral cavity is located on the anterior (front) side of the body. These cavities are almost completely sealed off from the external environment by surrounding bone and/or muscle and other connective tissue.

The dorsal cavity is subdivided into two main cavities: the cranial cavity and the vertebral or spinal cavity. The cranial cavity is located in the skull and encloses the brain, while the vertebral cavity is located within the spinal column and encloses the spinal cord. The dorsal cavity is lined with a layer of connective tissue called the meninges, which helps protect the delicate structures inside. It is also filled with cerebrospinal fluid, which acts as a cushion for the brain and spinal cord.

The dorsal cavity plays a crucial role in protecting and supporting the central nervous system, which is responsible for coordinating and controlling many of the body's functions. Any damage or injury to this area can result in serious consequences, including paralysis, loss of sensation, and even death.

The Ventral Cavity

The ventral cavity is a body cavity located on the anterior (front) side of the human body. The ventral cavity is larger and more complex than the dorsal cavity. It is enclosed by the inner walls of the thorax (i.e., thoracic muscles, ribs sternum, and thoracic vertebrae); the inner surfaces of the ventral, lateral, and dorsal abdominal wall muscles; and the inner surface bones and associated muscles of the pelvis.

The ventral cavity is divided into an upper cavity (thoracic cavity) and a lower cavity (abdominopelvic cavity) by a transverse dome-shaped muscle, the diaphragm. The thoracic cavity is located in the chest and contains the heart, lungs, and other structures of the respiratory and cardiovascular systems. The abdominopelvic cavity is located in the abdomen and pelvis and contains the digestive organs, reproductive organs, urinary system, and other structures.

The ventral cavity is lined with a thin layer of connective tissue called the serous membrane, which helps to protect and support the organs inside. This membrane produces a lubricating fluid that allows the organs to move against each other without causing friction or damage.

The ventral cavity plays a crucial role in maintaining the health and well-being of the body by containing and protecting many vital organs and systems. Any damage or injury to this area can have serious consequences, including respiratory failure, heart failure, organ failure, and other life-threatening conditions.

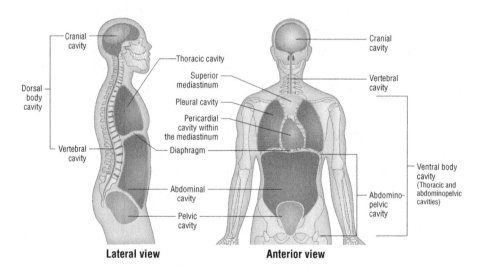

Lateral view   Anterior view

SKELETAL SYSTEM

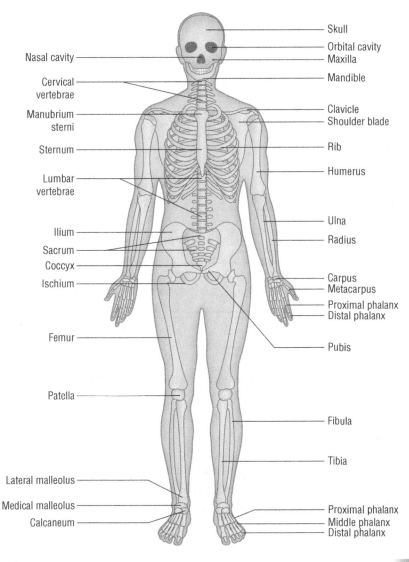

Skull

Orbital cavity

Nasal cavity

Maxilla

Mandible

Cervical vertebrae

Clavicle

Shoulder blade

Manubrium sterni

Rib

Sternum

Humerus

Lumbar vertebrae

Ulna

Ilium

Radius

Sacrum

Coccyx

Ischium

Carpus

Metacarpus

Proximal phalanx

Distal phalanx

Femur

Pubis

Patella

Fibula

Tibia

Lateral malleolus

Medical malleolus

Calcaneum

Proximal phalanx

Middle phalanx

Distal phalanx

Root Word	Meaning	Example
Oste(o)-	bone	osteitis, osteoma, osteocyte
Chondr(o)-	cartilage	chondritis, chondroma, chondrocyte
Arthr(o)-	joint	arthritis, arthroplasty
Myel(o)-	bone marrow	myeloma
Ten(o)-, Tendin(o)-	tendon (binds muscle to bone)	tendonitis, tenorrhaphy
Ligament(o)-	ligament (binds bone to bone)	ligamentous injury
Burs(o)-	bursa, bag (shock absorber between tendons and bones)	bursitis
My(o)-, Myos(o)-	muscle	myoma, myositis
-malacia	softening	osteomalacia, chondromalacia
-porosis	porous	osteoporosis
-asthenia	weakness, loss of strength	myasthenia gravis
-trophy	development, stimulation, maintenance	atrophy (shriveling of muscles), hypertrophy (increase in size and strength of muscles)

The Axial Skeleton

The axial skeleton consists of the bones of the skull and the spinal column, the ribs, and the sternum.

The Spine

In many respects, the spine is the fundamental structure of the human body. The spine consists of individual bones known as vertebrae arranged linearly to form a continuous, flexible, bony column.

The Vertebral Canal

The surfaces and underlying sub-regions of the spine and the individual verte-brae are the dorsal, ventral, lateral, and central regions. The central vertebral-spi-nal region is hollow and forms the vertebral canal. The vertebral canal contains the spinal cord of the central nervous system. The spinal cord begins as the distal extension of the brainstem and enters the vertebral canal through the fora-men magnum, a large opening in the posterior base of the skull.

The spinal cord does not extend for the entire length of the vertebral canal. Instead, the spinal cord terminates distally (or caudally) at the junction level of the first and second lumbar vertebrae. The dorsal and ventral spinal nerve roots that combine to form the 31 sets of spinal nerves of the somatic or voluntary nervous system emerge from the spinal cord at the dorsolateral and ventrolat-eral intervertebral junctions in the cervical, thoracic, and lumbar spinal regions.

The Skull

The skull consists of tightly fused bones that form the cranial vault and the facial bones. The cranial vault contains the brain and pituitary gland, and the facial bones include the upper jaw bones (i.e., the maxillae) and the lower jaw (i.e., the mandible). The mandible is the only moveable bone of the skull. The inner sur-faces of the bones that form the cranial cavity (cranial vault) correspond to the adjacent underlying regions of the cerebral cortex of the brain. The frontal bone overlies the left and right frontal cortices. The midline parietal bones overlie the parietal cortices. The laterally positioned temporal bones overlie the temporal cortices and the posteriorly positioned occipital bones form the back of the skull and overlie the occipital cortices.

The cerebellum and brainstem of the brain also occupy the occipital region of the cranial cavity at the base of the brain. A small depression called the sella turcica is in the media anterior inner surface of the base of the skull. Within the sella turcica, the pituitary gland is partially contained. The 12 pairs of cranial nerves emerge from the brain through various openings in the skull. Together with the 31 pairs of spinal nerves, these cranial nerves and spinal nerves form the somatic nervous system.

The Thoracic Skeleton

The thoracic (chest and upper back) skeleton comprises the thoracic vertebrae, 12 sets of ribs, the sternum (breastbone), and the medial sections of the clavicles (collarbones). The ribs connect to the lateral surfaces of the thoracic vertebrae and then extend laterally to form the dorsal thorax. Next, the ribs first curve anteriorly to form the lateral walls of the thorax and then curve medially, continuing to medially articulate with the sternum. The sternum is in the midline of the anterior (ventral) wall of the thorax. The medial ends of the clavicles articulate to the superolateral angles of the sternum.

The thoracic skeleton creates a cage-like structural framework. When the associated muscles and connective tissues are added to this framework, an interior thoracic cavity is created. This cavity contains the heart, lungs, and several other important anatomical structures. The floor of the thoracic cavity is formed via a single dome-shaped sheet of muscle, the diaphragm.

The Appendicular Skeleton

The upper appendicular (attached) skeleton consists of the bones of the shoulder girdles, arms, wrists, hands, and fingers. The shoulder girdles are formed by the clavicles and the scapulae. The medial ends of the clavicles articulate with the superolateral angles of the sternum. This connection is the only direct bony connection of the upper appendicular skeleton to the axial skeleton. The distal end of the scapula and a lateral extension of the clavicle (the acromion) articulate distally and, along with the proximal end of the humerus, forms the bony elements of the rotator cuff, the complex shoulder joint.

The distal end of the long bone of the upper arm (the humerus) forms the elbow joint with the proximal ends of the two lower arm bones, the radius and the ulna. The distal ends of the radius and the ulna articulate with several of the wrist bones (the carpals) to form the complex wrist joint. The carpals articulate with the metacarpal bones of the hand. The distal ends of the metacarpals articulate with the bones of the fingers, the phalanges.

The lower appendicular skeleton consists of the bones of the pelvis (except for the sacrum, which is part of the axial skeleton), and the bones of the legs, ankles, feet, and toes. The left and right portions of the bony pelvis are fused to the axial skeleton medially at the lateral edges of the sacrum. The proximal end or "head" of the femur fits into a semicircular depression of the inferolateral borders in the bones of the pelvis. Along with associated muscles and connective tissues, they form the ball and socket joint of the hip. The distal end of the femur articulates with the proximal ends of the tibia and fibula at the knee joint. The distal ends of the tibia and fibula articulate with several tarsal bones to form the complex ankle joint. Tarsal bones in the ankle region articulate with proximal ends of metatarsal bones in the foot. Distal ends of metatarsal bones articulate with the bones of the toes, the phalanges.

Skeletal Muscles

The skeletal structure of the body is mostly covered by layers of muscles. The anterior surface of the tibiae or shins and the wrists, ankles, cranium, and dorsal surface of the spine the ribs and the sternum and the clavicles have comparatively thin or extremely thin overlying layers of muscles. Major skeletal muscle groups include the following:

- Upper arm muscles, the biceps and triceps
- Deltoid muscles of the shoulders
- Large muscles of the anterior chest, the pectoralis major muscles
- Large lateral muscles of the back, the latissimus dorsi
- Large muscles of the pelvis (hips), the gluteal muscles
- Anterior muscles of the upper leg, the quadriceps
- Large muscles of the posterior upper leg, the hamstrings
- Largest muscles of the lower leg, the gastrocnemius (calf) muscles.

Synovial Joints

The adult human body has 206 major bones and many other smaller bones called sesamoid bones. Nearly all the major bones form articulations with adjacent bones (the patellae and the hyoid bone are notable exceptions). The widest range of motion occurs at synovial joints, which consist of a fibrous joint capsule that encloses the ends of two articulating bones. Ligaments between the articulating bone ends surround the exterior of the fibrous capsule and bind together the joint. The ends of the bones within the joint capsule are covered by pads of cartilage called articular cartilage, which provides mechanical protection to the ends of the bone; the pads are also slippery, allowing for ease of movement for bones within the synovial capsule.

Synovial Fluid

The interior surfaces of the synovial capsule are covered with specialized connective tissue that forms a synovial membrane. Fibroblasts within the synovial membrane secrete components of synovial fluid. These contributions to synovial fluid consist of long-chain sugar polymer molecules called hyaluronic acid and another molecule called lubrin. Both hyaluronic acid and lubrin provide lubrication to the joint structures within the synovial capsule. Additional elements of synovial fluid include water and dissolved oxygen and nutrients that diffuse from the capillaries within the synovial capsule.

Fibrous Joints and Sutures

Compared to synovial joints, fibrous joints are much simpler in structure. Fibrous joints consist of varying proportions of cartilage and/or collagen and elastic fibers; such joints allow very limited mobility. Fibrous joints are typically located between the edges of two adjacent bones, forming a seam between the bone borders like the mortar between bricks or masonry stones. Joint movement is limited to hinge-like flexion and extension at the fibrous seam between adjacent bone edges. The sternomanubrial joint and the sacroiliac joints are fibrous joints that have a moderated amount of flexibility. Suture joints, which have very little fibrous content and almost no range of motion, are the strongest joints and are analogous to seam welds between adjacent bone edges. The bones of the skull (except for the mandible) articulate with suture joints.

Bone Classification by Shape

The bones of the human body can be classified by shape into one of five general categories: long bones, short bones, flat bones, irregular bones, and sesamoid bones.

Long Bones

Long bones have a tubular shape with a long axis several times greater than a cross-sectional diameter. The longest section of long bones is the bone shaft or diaphysis. The ends of long bones are called epiphyses. They are located at either end of the shaft (diaphysis) and have expanded and often complex geometries beautifully designed to allow the types of motion that occur when the long bones articulate with adjacent epiphyses within a synovial joint. The major bones of the upper and lower arms and legs (the humerus, femur, radius, ulna, tibia, and fibula) are long bones. The phalanges (finger and toe bones) and the clavicles (collarbones) are also long bones. Most long bones have medullary cavities and are a major site of erythropoiesis.

Epiphyseal plates

The cartilaginous epiphyseal plates of the upper and lower extremities are a primary site for growth resulting in increased bone length. The adult height of an individual is determined by the amount of growth that occurs at the epiphyseal plates of these long bones and in the vertebrae of the spine. When the cartilage of the epiphyseal plates of long bones and vertebrae become fully mineralized into bone, no further increase in height can occur in an individual. The closure of these epiphyseal plates is a primary indication that an individual has reach adulthood.

Short Bones

Short bones have variable shapes, often cuboidal with dimensions of roughly equivalent length, width, and height.

The wrist and ankle bones

The bones of the wrists and ankles (metacarpals and the metatarsals, respectively) and the middle bones of the hands and feet (the carpals and tarsals, respectively) are short bones. Each hand has eight carpal bones; each foot has seven tarsal bones. These bones are closely packed and have multiple interfaces with adjacent carpals or tarsals. At the ankle and wrist, for example, some tarsal or carpal bones articulate with metacarpals or metatarsals.

Metacarpals and metatarsals also articulate with adjacent long bone epiphyses of the radius and ulna, or the tibia and fibula. In addition, some tarsals and carpals articulate with epiphyses of phalanges in the hands to form the "knuckle" joints.

Due to multiple articulations with adjacent bones, carpals, metacarpals, tarsals, and metatarsals tend to have complex surface geometry and irregular overall three-dimensional shapes. These bones are designed to function as a group of subunits that allow for very complex and subtle rearrangements of the contours of the palms of the hands and soles of the feet. These continuous alterations in the contours of the palms and soles are required particularly when walking on uneven surfaces or when grasping and manipulating objects. While these multi-bone systems allow for remarkable adaptability during walking and running activities and exceptional dexterity of the hands, even seemingly minor injuries to an individual ankle or wrist bone can destabilize the entire wrist or ankle system, leading to severe impairment of function.

Irregular Bones

As a general category, irregular bones have complex three dimensional geometries. The range of irregularity varies greatly, however. By far the most irregular bones are two of the skull bones, the vomer and the sphenoid bones. These bones have complex three-dimensional overall and local structures consisting of bony walls, partitions, shelves, protuberances, compartments, passageways, and openings that accommodate a variety of contents. For example, the sphenoid is particularly designed for a broad range of structural and functional purposes. Many anatomists have opined that the sphenoid is a bone whose structure is so complex that "it defies description." Several other bones of the cranium and the face are irregular bones or have irregular regions. For example: the ethmoid, mastoid, and maxillary bones. The bones of the pelvis (the ilium, ischium pubis, and sacroiliac bones) are also irregular bones.

The bones of the middle ear—the incus, malleus, and stapes (anvil, hammer, and stirrup)—are irregular in the sense of not having a simple shape, but they each have a very specific shape that allows them to function together as a unit. These three middle ear bones form a linked bony mechanical system that transduces sound waves arriving at the tympanum (eardrum) in the outer ear canal to fluid waves within the canals of the inner ear.

The spinal vertebrae

The individual vertebrae of the spine are classified as irregular bones but are comparable in structure and in articulations with adjacent vertebrae to the short bones of the ankle and wrists. The "irregularity" of the vertebrae consists of their vertebral foramen, left and right transverse processes, and dorsal midline single spinous processes.

The central canal of a vertebra is a tubular passage that aligns with the vertebral foramen of adjacent vertebrae. In the spine, these central canals form a continuous tube called the spinal canal. The spinal cord is contained within the spinal canal. The dorsal spinous process of a vertebra is a single long projection of the dorsal surface of a vertebra. The tips of spinous processes can, as a group, be seen and felt as the longitudinal arrangement of bumps that define the location of spine underlying the skin in the midline of the dorsal surface of the torso.

These additional features of a vertebrae are very regular and differ slightly but regularly between vertebrae, primarily in the length and thickness of the spinous processes in the cervical, thoracic, and lumbar sections of the spine and in the mass of the main body of the vertebrae, from smallest at the first cervical vertebrae (CI and C2) to largest at the most caudal lumbar vertebrae (L4 and LS). The vertebrae function as subunits of the overall spine. Although the range of motion between adjacent vertebrae is limited, when coordinated along the length of the spine, these motions can cumulatively produce a remarkable range of bending and twisting spinal movements. As a result, the human body can adopt a vast number of specific postures in three dimensions and coordinate changing postures to create complex, dynamic choreographies of continuous body movements.

Intervertebral discs

A unique feature of the spinal vertebrae is the intervertebral discs. These are shock-absorbing structures consisting of a tough outer fibrous capsule that encases a gel-like substance called the nucleus pulposus. The discs act as a fibrocartilaginous joint between adjacent vertebrae.

Flat Bones and Sesamoid Bones

Flat bones are thin with a high surface area. They have an outer layer of cortical bone and a thin central layer of trabecular bone. In the cranium, most bones are flat bones. Flat bones have a primary protective function—particularly the protection of the brain—and have little if any role in erythropoiesis.

On the other hand, sesamoid bones are formed with muscle tendons and have a mechanical function related to the amount of leverage that a muscle can generate on an attached bone. Most sesamoid bones are relatively small; a notable exception is the patella, which is located anterior to the synovial joint of the knee.

Bone and Joint Disorders

Many diseases and other pathological conditions of bones and joints are notable for the frequency and/or severity in humans. Joint disorders are so common that one medical specialty—rheumatology—focuses exclusively on the diagnosis and treatment of these conditions.

Disorders of the Synovial Joints

The two most important synovial joint disorders are rheumatoid arthritis and osteoarthritis. Rheumatoid arthritis is an autoimmune disorder that attacks synovial joints, resulting in progressive, painful disfigurement and loss of function in joints throughout the body. Modern treatment involves monoclonal antibodies and other immunological therapies that can prevent the progression of the disease if the condition is diagnosed in its early stages.

Osteoarthritis is a result of the wear-and-tear damage to the articular cartilage in synovial joints. The mechanical forces acting on joints over decades of physical activity eventually wear away the cartilage in synovial joints, resulting in the loss of the protection the cartilage provides to underlying bone. The unprotected articulating bones grind against each other and cause severe pain and eventually loss of function. Most middle-aged to elderly males have some degree of osteoarthritis. The condition is most serious when the knee and hip joints are involved. In the United States, damage due to osteoarthritis is the number one reason for hip and knee replacements.

Infection, Inflammation, and Physical Injury

Synovial fluid is susceptible to accumulations of uric acid crystals, resulting in the excruciatingly painful inflammatory condition known as gout. Bacteria that enter the bloodstream often settle in synovial joints and cause infection or septic arthritis. Many viral and autoimmune diseases also attack synovial joints and cause sterile or aseptic arthritis. The joints are common sites of severe physical injuries, including ligament and tendon tears and ruptures, and joint sprains and dislocations. The deep tendon reflexes are a specialized local neuromuscular reflex that has evolved to limit such injuries.

A particularly significant class of joint disorders are those of the intervertebral discs. Herniated vertebral discs usually occur due to awkward and/or strenuous lifting and twisting activities. Degenerative disc disease (DJD) is a progressive deterioration of the intervertebral discs. Both conditions are very common; in fact, lower back pain associated with these disorders is one of the leading causes people seek medical attention.

Disorders of the Bone

Osteoporosis is the most common serious bone disorder and most commonly occurs in postmenopausal women. The condition is a loss of bone density and disruption of bone structure primarily due to inadequate calcium content. People with osteoporosis are at greatly increased risk of bone fractures, most seriously fractures of the pelvic bones or the femur. Estrogen replacement therapy in postmenopausal women can greatly reduce the incidence of osteoporosis, but this form of treatment must be balanced against the risks of the therapy, including increased risk of cardiovascular disease. Regular physical activity and weight-bearing exercise reduces the risk of osteoporosis.

Although rare in developed countries, rickets is a common bone disorder elsewhere. The disorder is caused by vitamin D deficiency. If left untreated, rickets results in deterioration of bone tissue; bones become increasingly brittle and fracture easily. Osteomalacia (vitamin D-resistant rickets), which causes a disease that resembles rickets, leads to not only bone weakness but also abnormal bone formation. The condition is the result of a defect in vitamin D metabolism.

Paget's disease is characterized by abnormal structural development, including enlargement and thickening of bones that are brittle and easily broken. The condition results from abnormalities of osteoblast and osteoclast functions.

Perthes' disease, which occurs primarily in children, is a disorder of the femoral head of the tibia at the ball-and-socket joint of the hip. The condition is caused by inadequate blood supply to the femoral head and results in pain and an impaired ability to walk or run.

Osteogenesis Imperfecta (brittle bone disease) is an autosomal dominant genetic disorder caused by defects in the enzymes involved in collagen production. The result is brittle bones that fracture easily.

Acromegaly is condition caused by an excess of growth hormone and continued growth hormone production after individuals have completed puberty. Most commonly, the abnormal growth hormone production is due to a benign tumor of the pituitary gland. If left untreated, acromegaly results in progressive enlargement of the facial, hand, and feet bones. This process can continue over the entire life of an individual.

Bone Marrow Disorders

Bone marrow suppression and bone marrow failure occur as a relatively common and often life-threatening condition. The hematopoietic cells of bone marrow are particularly sensitive to a wide variety of drugs, including antibiotics, anti-inflammatories, anti-cancer drugs, and many other commonly used drugs. Bone marrow cells are also easily damaged by environmental toxins, such as cleaning agents, heavy metals, and insecticides and herbicides. In addition, bone marrow is very vulnerable to radiation-induced injuries from medical and dental x-ray imagery and from artificial and naturally occurring radioactive compounds in the environment.

As these conditions worsen and persist, the granulocytes and lymphocyte cell production drop or even cease, resulting in profound impairment of the immune system. Impaired red cell production results in severe anemia, and impaired platelet production results in spontaneous hemorrhages. All these effects can be rapidly fatal if not corrected promptly. Most blood cancers, including leukemias and lymphomas, originate from abnormal cells in the bone marrow.

MUSCULAR SYSTEM

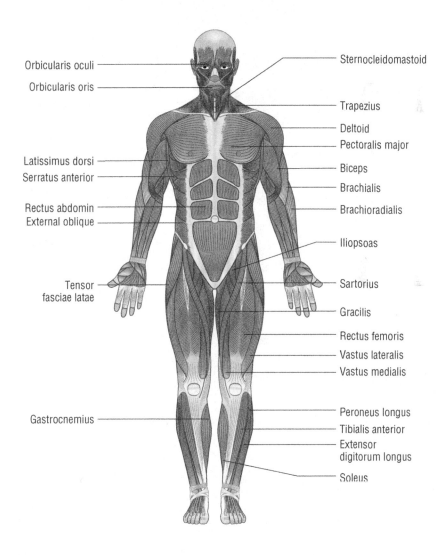

Orbicularis oculi

Orbicularis oris

Latissimus dorsi

Serratus anterior

Rectus abdomin

External oblique

Tensor
fasciae latae

Gastrocnemius

Sternocleidomastoid

Trapezius

Deltoid

Pectoralis major

Biceps

Brachialis

Brachioradialis

Iliopsoas

Sartorius

Gracilis

Rectus femoris

Vastus lateralis

Vastus medialis

Peroneus longus

Tibialis anterior

Extensor
digitorum longus

Soleus

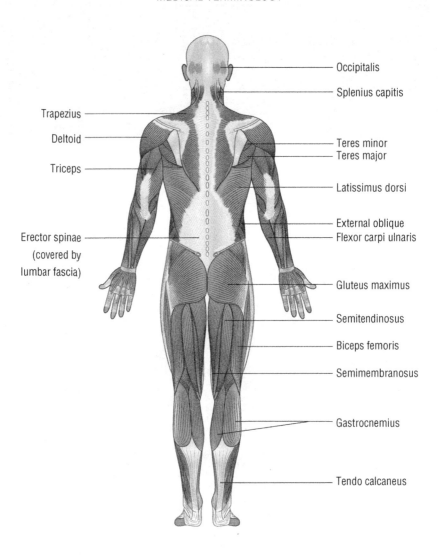

Occipitalis

Splenius capitis

Trapezius

Deltoid

Teres minor

Teres major

Triceps

Latissimus dorsi

External oblique

Flexor carpi ulnaris

Erector spinae
(covered by
lumbar fascia)

Gluteus maximus

Semitendinosus

Biceps femoris

Semimembranosus

Gastrocnemius

Tendo calcaneus

Root Word	Meaning	Examples
Oste(o)-	bone	osteitis, osteoma, osteocyte
Chondr(o)-	cartilage	chondritis, chondroma, chondrocyte
Arthr(o)-	joint	arthritis, arthroplasty
Myel(o)-	bone marrow	myeloma
Ten(o)-, Tendin(o)-	tenon (binds muscle to bone)	tendonitis, tenorrhaphy
Ligament(o)-	ligament (binds bone to bone)	ligamentous injury
Burs/o-	bursa, bag (shock absorber between tendons and bones)	bursitis
My(o)-, Myos(o)-	muscle	myoma, myositis
-malacia	softening	osteomalacia, chondromalacia
-porosis	porous	osteoporosis
-asthenia	weakness, loss of strength	myasthenia gravis
-trophy	development, stimulation, maintenance	atrophy (shriveling of muscles), hypertrophy (increase in size and strength of muscles)
-algia, -algesia	pain	myalgia, arthralgia, analgesia (inability to feel pain.)

Most of the body skeletal structure body is covered by layers of muscles. Areas of the body that have comparatively thin or extremely thin overlying layers of muscles include: the anterior surface of the tibiae or shins; the wrists, ankles, cranium, and dorsal surface of the spine; the ribs and the sternum; and the clavicles.

The muscular system is composed of muscle fibers. Muscle fiber's main function is to contract and enable movement (contractility). Almost all movement in the body is caused by muscle contraction. To move the skeletal bones, the muscle fibers contact, create tension, and the tension is transferred to the tendons (which are strong bands of dense connective tissue that connect muscles to bones), and then to then to the periosteum to pull on the bone for movement of the skeleton. When not contracting, a muscle can relax and revert to its original length (elasticity). Muscle tissue can also stretch or extend (extensibility). Contractility, elasticity, and extensibility make muscle one of the most versatile tissue types of the human body.,

Skeletal muscles do not work by in isolation. Instead, they are attached to the bones of the skeleton in pairs. The integrated action of tendons, joints, bones, and skeletal muscles enables movements such as lifting, walking, and running, or other more subtle movements such as facial expressions. Muscle contraction also helps maintain body posture, joint stability, and is largely responsible for the body's heat production.

Major Muscle Groups

Major skeletal muscle groups include the following groups:

- Upper arm muscles, the biceps and triceps
- Deltoid muscles of the shoulders
- Large muscles of the anterior chest the pectoralis major muscles
- Large lateral muscles of the back, the latissimus dorsi
- Large muscles of the pelvis (hips), the gluteal muscles
- Anterior muscles of the upper leg, the quadriceps
- Large muscles of the posterior upper leg, the hamstrings
- Largest muscle of the lower leg, the gastrocnemius (calf) muscles

Muscle Naming Conventions

A skeletal muscle is oftentimes named after its distinguishing features. Here is a list of such features, followed by examples:

- Anatomical location or relationship to the bone(s) a muscle is attached to: temporalis, which is in the temple area and attached to the temporal bone; pectoralis (chest); gluteus (buttock); brachii (arm); lateralis (lateral).

- Position relative to the body midline: medialis (toward the midline); lateralis (towards the outside and away from the midline).
- Shape of the muscle: orbicularis (the Latin root word "orbiculus" means "small disk"); deltoid (triangular); rhomboid (like a rhombus with equal and parallel sides).
- Size of the muscle: gluteus minimus; gluteus maximus; gluteus medius.
- Length of the muscle—brevis (short), longus (long): peroneus Brevis; adductor longus.
- Movement produced by the muscle—flexor, extensor, abductor, adductor, levator: flexor pollicis longus; adductor longus; adductor magnus.
- Direction of the muscle fibers and fascicles: external oblique of the abdomen; rectus (straight) abdominis.
- Number of muscles in a group or origins a muscle has: biceps; triceps; quadriceps.

Muscle Types

The three types of muscle are skeletal, smooth, and cardiac.

Skeletal muscle

Skeletal muscle is attached to bones, its contraction produces skeletal movements, facial expressions, posture, and other voluntary movements of the body. The peripheral portion of the central nervous system controls the skeletal muscles. Skeletal muscle cells have many nuclei squeezed along the membranes. Skeletal muscle fibers are striated with transverse streaks. The striation can be attributed to: 1) the regular alternation of the contractile proteins actin and myosin; and 2) the structural proteins that couple the contractile proteins to connective tissues. Skeletal muscle fibers act independently of neighboring muscle fibers.

Skeletal muscles not only enable body movements, but they also contribute to the maintenance of homeostasis by generating heat. Skeletal muscle is richly supplied by blood vessels for nutrition supply, oxygen delivery, and waste removal.

The energy supply required for muscle contraction is produced through breaking down ATP, and heat is generated in this process as a byproduct. Such heat production is very noticeable during physical activity. During low temperature, the body's involuntary shivering produces heat to maintain body temperature.

Skeletal muscle fiber is also supplied by the axon branch of a somatic motor neuron, which controls the contraction and relaxation of muscle fiber. Under the conscious control of the central nervous system, skeletal muscles initiate movement, stop movement, maintain posture and balance. Muscles also maintain skeletal and joint stability and integrity by preventing excess movement of the bones and joints. Muscles located throughout the body, such as the genioglossus muscle, styloglossus muscle, urethral sphincter, and anal sphincter, also help control basic bodily functions such as food intake, urination, and defecation.

Smooth muscle

Smooth muscle is in the walls of the hollow internal organs such as blood vessels, the gastrointestinal tract, bladder, uterus, reproductive systems, and the airways. Smooth muscle is under control of the autonomic nervous system and its contraction cannot be controlled consciously. The non-striated (smooth) muscle cell is spindle-shaped, with a single central nucleus. Smooth muscle contracts slowly and rhythmically.

Cardiac muscle

Cardiac muscle forms the contractile walls of the heart. It is under the control of the autonomic nervous system and cannot be controlled consciously. The cells of cardiac muscle, known as cardiomyocytes, are striated, like those of the skeletal muscle fiber. However, unlike skeletal muscle fibers, cardiomyocytes are single cells that typically have a single nucleus that resembles that of the smooth muscle. The contraction of cardiac muscle is strong and rhythmical. A mechanical and electrochemical syncytium allows the cardiac cells to synchronize their contractions and relaxations.

CARDIOVASCULAR SYSTEM

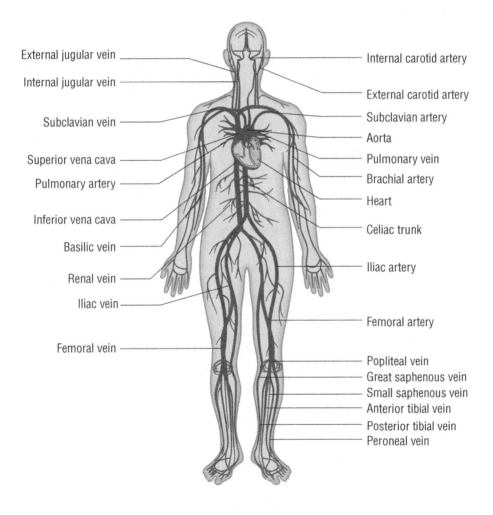

External jugular vein

Internal jugular vein

Subclavian vein

Superior vena cava

Pulmonary artery

Inferior vena cava

Basilic vein

Renal vein

Iliac vein

Femoral vein

Internal carotid artery

External carotid artery

Subclavian artery

Aorta

Pulmonary vein

Brachial artery

Heart

Celiac trunk

Iliac artery

Femoral artery

Popliteal vein

Great saphenous vein

Small saphenous vein

Anterior tibial vein

Posterior tibial vein

Peroneal vein

Root Word	Meaning	Examples
Cardi(o)-	heart	endocarditis, myocarditis, pericarditis (inflammation of the lining, the muscle layer, the outer layer of the heart)
Brady-, Tachy-	slow/fast	bradycardia (rate<60) tachycardia (rate>100)
Angi(o)-,	vessel	angiography, angiogram (x-ray of artery)
Veno-, Phlebo-	vein	venogram (x-ray of veins), phlebitis (inflammation of veins)
-stasis	to stop	hemostasis (to stop bleeding), hemostat (a clamp-like instrument)
-cyte	cell	erythrocytes, leukocytes (red, white blood cells)
Hem(o)-, -emia	blood	hypoxemia (low oxygen), hematosalpinx (blood in the uterine tubes)

The anatomy of the cardiovascular circulatory system begins with the heart, located at the base of the thoracic cavity directly superior to the diaphragm and centered slightly left of the midline of the sternum. The lower lobes of the left and right lungs are immediately lateral to the lateral walls of the heart.

The heart consists of muscular walls that enclose four chambers: the thin-walled right and left atria, and the thick-walled right and left ventricles. The right and left ventricles share a common medial wall (interventricular septum), as do the right and left atria (interatrial septum). The right atrium is directly superior to the right ventricle, and the left atrium is directly superior to the left ventricle. The atria and ventricles are separated by a common septum (atrioventricular septum), which forms the bases or floors of the atria and the ceilings of the underling ventricles of each atrium.

Cardiovascular Blood Flow

Deoxygenated blood from all other body regions arrives at the heart via veins. The smaller veins eventually pass blood through to either the superior or inferior vena cava, the largest veins of the body. The superior and inferior vena cava both empty into the right atrium. Blood then passes from the right atrium through a three-leaflet valve (the tricuspid valve) into the right ventricle. Subsequently, this blood is pumped out the right ventricle through a two-leaflet valve (the pulmonic valve) into the main pulmonary artery. Blood in the main pulmonary artery continues to either the left or right pulmonary arteries, which then enter either the left or the right lung.

Pulmonary Blood Flow

The pulmonary arteries branch into increasingly smaller and more numerous arteries. The smallest terminal arterial branches are the arterioles. From the arterioles, blood passes into capillaries (one-cell thick walled vessels). Blood passing through these capillaries exchanges oxygen from inspired (inhaled) air in alveolar airspaces. Carbon dioxide diffuses from the blood in the capillaries and into the alveolar airspaces before being expelled from the body via respiratory airways during exhalation (expiration).

The capillary blood, now oxygenated, passes first to venules, then to larger veins, and finally returns to the heart via the main pulmonary veins. The main pulmonary veins (usually four these) empty into the left atrium. Blood from the left atrium passes into the left ventricle through a two-leaflet valve (the mitral valve). The blood is then pumped from the heart via the left ventricle through a two-leaflet valve (the aortic valve) into the aorta.

The aorta is the largest artery in the body. From the aorta, oxygenated blood is delivered through a network of branching arterial trees to all regions of the body. Oxygen and nutrients are transferred to tissues, and carbon dioxide and other waste products are absorbed in capillary beds, which refers to the interweaving network of capillaries supplying tissues and organs. Capillary blood, now deoxygenated, returns to the heart via networks of veins, as already described.

Portal Vein Systems

An important anatomical concept in the cardiovascular system is that blood pumped away from the heart, either via the left or the right ventricle, always first enters a main artery, then travels to sequentially smaller arteries, then travels to the smallest arteries (arterioles), and finally enters capillaries. From the capillaries, this blood travels to the smallest veins (venules), and then to the larger veins. Most of this blood travels to sequentially larger veins and directly back to the heart, but some of the blood is routed through a second set of capillary beds. Most notably, the latter occurs with venous blood traveling from capillary beds in the intestines to capillary beds in the liver. This type of circulatory anatomy is classified as a "portal system" or "portal circulation."

Cardiovascular (Circulatory) Physiology

The primary functions of the cardiovascular system are (1) to deliver oxygen from the lungs to all the cells of the body along with water, electrolytes, glucose, and other essential substances, and (2) to transport waste products to the organs responsible for detoxifying and excreting waste products from the body. Carbon dioxide is delivered to the lungs, and other wastes are delivered either directly or indirectly to the kidneys through the liver. To accomplish these functions, the circulatory vessels must maintain a large, driving blood-pressure differential between the arterial side of the heart (the left heart) and the venous side of the heart (the right heart).

Mechanics of Cardiac Pressure and Blood Flow

The heart is a muscular organ composed primarily of cardiac muscle. The atria of the heart are thin-walled compared to the ventricles of the heart. This difference exists because the atria receive low pressure venous blood from the body and do not need to generate high blood pressure to pump blood to the ventricles. Comparatively, the ventricles are thick-walled and designed to generate high blood pressures that drive blood through the arterial vessels. The direction of blood flow within the heart is accomplished by the arrangement of one-way valves within the heart and the sequence in which various regions of the heart contract during a cardiac cycle.

Arteries

Arteries are designed to withstand the high pressure generated by the ventricles of the heart. Arteries must also be able to stretch when blood flow volumes increase greatly during ventricular contractions and contract to maintain adequate blood pressures in the intervals between ventricular contractions. This ability requires thick arterial walls with elastic protein fibers and a layer of smooth muscle cells.

Arterioles

As the arterial vasculature progresses from the heart, large arteries split into numerous branches of smaller diameter arteries. The final arterial branches are the arterioles. As the smallest diameter arteries, the arterioles connect to capillaries. The arteriole walls contain smooth muscles that can relax or contract in response to numerous types of stimuli, some local and some in the form of hormonal or electrical to signals from the nervous system. Arteriolar contraction can completely close off blood flow to capillary beds, and arteriolar relaxation increases blood flow to capillary beds. At this level, many body systems regulate blood distribution and organ function based on the needs of the body at any given time.

Capillaries

Capillaries are designed to maximize the diffusion of substances entering and leaving the circulatory system. This maximization is accomplished by minimizing the structures and distances that substances must cross when passing through capillary walls. To facilitate this process, capillaries are only one-cell layer in thickness.

Fluid Compartments of the Body

The body has three major fluid compartments: the intravascular space (space inside blood vessels and the heart; the extracellular space (space outside blood vessels, the heart, and all cells of the body); and the intracellular space (total space within all the cells of the body). Oxygen, nutrients, water, waste products, and all other water-soluble biological substances diffuse between the intravascular space and the extracellular space, and between the extracellular space and the intracellular space. Water diffuses freely between all three spaces; the distribution of water is determined by the osmolality of the fluid compartments. The major osmotic particles in fluid compartments are proteins, which do not diffuse across cell membranes that separate fluid compartments (except by active transport processes).When the arterioles feeding capillaries are open, the blood pressure within capillaries is higher than the fluid pressure in the extracellular compartment; this higher pressure drives water from the capillaries. The proteins in the blood inside capillaries limit the water loss from the intravascular space via osmotic pressure effects. Oxygen, nutrients, and other essential biological substances diffuse down concentration gradients from the capillaries and into the extravascular space. The reverse process occurs for waste products in the extracellular space.

Veins

Excess water is reabsorbed by lymphatic vessels and by the venules, the venous vessels at the other end of capillaries. Venules are the terminal branches of the venous side of the circulatory system. Veins return blood to the heart (except in portal systems). Venules converge on large veins and then to still larger veins, eventually converging into the superior and inferior vena cava. The blood pressure in veins is much lower than on the arterial side; consequently, veins are thin-walled since they are not subject to high arterial pressure. Venous blood flow from the extremities is greatly aided by skeletal muscle contractions and associated limb movements. Veins also have internal one-way valves that allow blood to flow freely toward the heart but prevent blood flow in the opposite direction (backflow).

NERVOUS SYSTEM

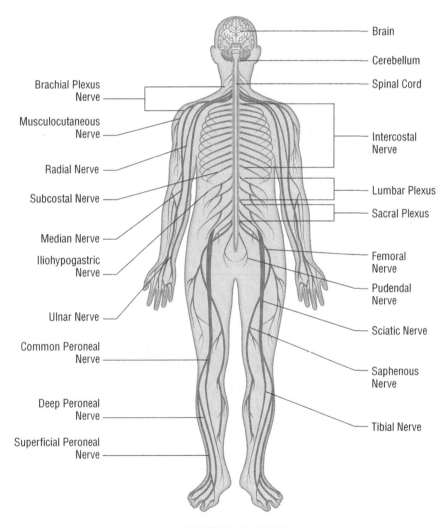

Brain

Cerebellum

Spinal Cord

Brachial Plexus Nerve

Musculocutaneous Nerve

Intercostal Nerve

Radial Nerve

Subcostal Nerve

Lumbar Plexus

Sacral Plexus

Median Nerve

Iliohypogastric Nerve

Femoral Nerve

Pudendal Nerve

Ulnar Nerve

Sciatic Nerve

Common Peroneal Nerve

Saphenous Nerve

Deep Peroneal Nerve

Superficial Peroneal Nerve

Tibial Nerve

NERVOUS SYSTEM

Root Word	Meaning	Examples
Cephal(o)-	head	cephalgia (a headache)
Encephal(o)-	inside the head (brain)	encephalitis (inflammation of the brain), anencephalic (born without a brain)
Mening(o)-	membranes surrounding the brain and spinal cord	meningitis (inflammation of the membranes)
Myel(o)-	spinal cord	myelogram (x-ray of the spinal cord)
Neur(o)-	nerve	neuroma (tumor) neuritis (inflammation)
Dys-	difficult, painful, abnormal	dyslexia (difficulty reading)
-cele	hernia, abnormal protrusion of structure outside the normal anatomical position	meningomyelocele (protrusion of membranes and spinal cord)
-pathy	disease, abnormality	encephalopathy (disease of the brain), neuropathy (disease of the nerves)
-plasia	development, formation, growth	aplasia (no development), hyperplasia (over development)
-plegia	paralysis	hemiplegia (paralysis of one side of the body), quadriplegia (paralysis of all four limbs)

The nervous system can be anatomically divided into the central nervous system and the peripheral nervous systems.

The Central Nervous System

The central nervous system, as previously noted, consists of the brain (in the cranial cavity) and the spinal cord (in the vertebral canal of the spine). Also mentioned was that the outermost or most superficial region of the terminal end of the brain, the cerebral cortex, consists of five regions or lobes. The frontal, parietal temporal, and occipital lobes underlie the cranial bones of the corresponding designations. The cerebral cortex is divided into two hemispheres, right and left, connected by large nerve tracts. The largest of these tracts is the corpus callosum. Each hemisphere consists of the five cerebral cortical lobes; thus, there are right and left frontal, parietal temporal, and occipital lobes.

The regions of the brain between the cerebral cortex and the spinal cord include the midbrain, the cerebellum, and the brainstem. The brainstem is continuous with the spinal cord as the spinal cord enters the brain at the base of the skull. More specific notable brain regions include the medulla oblongata (in the brainstem) and the hypothalamus (in the midbrain at the base of the skull). The pituitary gland is an important endocrine structure adjacent and inferior to the hypothalamus.

The spinal cord is the distal continuation of the brain stem and is contained within the vertebral canal. Beginning at the base of the occipital region of the skull, the spinal cord continues to its terminus at the junction of the first and second lumbar vertebrae. The spinal cord has relatively few neuron cell bodies, instead consistently of mainly nerves that relay information between the brain and neurons of the peripheral nervous system. The 31 pairs of spinal nerves exit the spinal cord at the interspaces between adjoining vertebrae, one pair per intervertebral junction.

The 12 pairs of cranial nerves and 31 pairs of spinal nerves become important elements of the peripheral nervous system once they have exited from the cranial or vertebral cavities.

The Peripheral Nervous System

The peripheral nervous system is the portion of the nervous system that lies outside the brain and spinal cord. It collects information from different areas of the body and delivers that information back to the brain; and it also carries out commands from the brain to various parts of the body. All elements of the nervous system—neurons, nerves (axons of neurons), sensory cells, effector cells (muscle cells and glands), and supporting cells and structures not located either inside the skull or the spinal column—are also elements of the peripheral nervous system.

It is important to understand that the distinction between the central nervous system and the peripheral nervous system is purely an anatomical one. All the neurological activity in the body is ultimately under the control of the central nervous system, and all the neurons in the peripheral nervous system have nerve pathways that connect to the brain.

Two broad divisions exist in the peripheral nervous system: (1) the voluntary or somatic nervous system and (2) the involuntary or autonomic nervous system.

The Somatic (Voluntary) Nervous System

The somatic nervous system, as previously mentioned, consists of 12 pairs of cranial nerves and 31 pairs of spinal nerves. These nerves carry sensory information from sensory receptor cells located throughout the body to the brain. The nerves also carry instructions, in the form of electrical impulses, from the brain to effector cells located throughout the body. In most cases, the effector cells are skeletal muscle cells or glands (endocrine and exocrine glands). The sensory information provided by the peripheral nervous system is integrated with other conscious thought processes and allow people to make voluntary decisions to complete physical actions. These decisions are translated into actions, starting with the generation and transmission of electrical signals through the somatic nerves to skeletal muscles. Skeletal muscles relax and contract in a way that results in the desired body movements. Often, these highly complex movements occur in the muscles of the vocal cords to produce speech.

Somatic ganglia

An important anatomical feature of the somatic nervous system is that the spinal peripheral nerves originate from collections of neuron cell bodies in discrete regions of the vertebrae but outside the vertebral canal. Collections of neuron cell bodies not inside the central nervous system are classified as "ganglia." The sensory ganglia are found in the dorsal regions of vertebrae and are called dorsal root ganglia. Neurons in the dorsal ganglia contribute the sensory nerve fibers to spinal nerves. In ventral regions of the vertebrae, ventral root ganglia neurons contribute the nerve fibers that send signals to effector cells. These types of nerves are called motor nerves.

The Autonomic (Involuntary) Nervous System

Most of the neural regulatory activity of the body is not under voluntary control. The central nervous system regulates most body functions through the involuntary or autonomic nervous system. The two divisions of the autonomic nervous system are the sympathetic and the parasympathetic nervous systems. These systems are commonly described as the "fight or flight" nervous system (sympathetic division) and the "rest and digest" nervous system (parasympathetic division). Again, realizing both systems are directly connected to specific regions of the brain is important. The systems are not an independent peripheral nervous system. Rather, they have an extensive peripheral component and a highly complex central component.

One notable general anatomical feature is that the autonomic nerve fibers are usually not organized into separate specific nerves, but often are nerve fibers that follow the course of and may even be adherent to blood vessels or somatic nerves.

The Sympathetic Nervous System

The peripheral component of the sympathetic nervous system begins with the neuron cell bodies in the sympathetic ganglia. Most of these ganglia are in pairs just lateral to the spinal cord and are therefore often referred to as the sympathetic "chain" ganglia. These ganglia send nerve fibers throughout the body, particularly to the organs, glands, and blood vessels of the body.

The Parasympathetic Nervous System

The peripheral component of the parasympathetic nervous system begins with the neuron cell bodies in the parasympathetic ganglia. In contrast to the sympathetic ganglia, the parasympathetic ganglia are usually located close to the organs and local anatomic regions that they innervate (supply nerves to). The Vagus nerve or 10th (X) cranial nerve is particularly important in the parasympathetic nervous system. This nerve carries parasympathetic nerve fibers to most of the major organs of the body, including the heart, the lungs, and much of the digestive system.

Neurophysiology

Nervous tissue consists of two types of cells, neurons and glial cells. Neurons are responsible for the computation and communication functions of the nervous system. They can send electrical and chemical signals to target cells. Glial cells, or glia, play a supporting role for the nervous tissue.

Neurons

At the cellular level, the production, transmission, and processing or integration of information in the form of electrical impulses is carried out by neurons. Neurons are electrically excitable cells (muscle cells are also electrically excitable cells). All cells in the body maintain concentration levels of ions inside the cell (particularly for Na+, K+, Na+, and Cl) that are different than the ion concentrations outside the cell. This difference of ion concentrations causes a voltage difference across the cell membrane.

Electrically excitable cells have specialized membrane pores and ion pumps that can use this voltage difference to generate a voltage spike called an action potential, which travels along the cell membrane.

Axons, Dendrites, and Synapses

The neuron has, in most cases, a very long membrane extension called the axon, which looks like a tail. The nerves of the body comprise these neuron axons. The sciatic nerve, which extends from the spine to the toes, can consist of numerous individual neuron axons, each several feet in length. Action potentials generated by the neuron at the base of the axon travel along the axon to its terminal end.

At the end of the axon, a dendrite (a branch-like extension of another neuron) is usually found. The action potential in the first neuron axon causes the release of neurotransmitters, which are small molecules that diffuse across the gap between the axon and the dendrite of the second neuron. The neurotransmitter molecules bind to receptors on the second neuron's dendritic membrane. This binding can cause the second neuron to generate its own action potential, which again travels down the second neuron's axon.

Through this method, electrical impulses can be transmitted from one neuron to another. The location at which the diffusion of neurotransmitters between two neurons occurs is called a synapse. The human brain has more than an estimated 100 trillion synapses.

The Medulla Oblongata

Among the most ancient regions of the brain, the medulla oblongata is in the brainstem adjacent to the spinal cord. The medulla is responsible for maintaining heart rate, breathing rate, and blood pressure, but plays other key roles in the homeostatic control of all body systems.

The Hypothalamus

A midbrain structure located at the base of the skull, the hypothalamus is a critical region in homeostatic regulation. The hypothalamus either directly or indirectly detects blood pH and osmolality levels, oxygen levels, and numerous other biochemical and physiological metrics. Most of the drive state sensations—including hunger, thirst, and excessive heat and cold—are generated by the hypothalamus. The hypothalamus is integrated with other brain regions to respond to homeostatic needs via activation of the sympathetic and parasympathetic nervous system, and through the secretion of hypothalamic hormones that directly influence the activity of all other endocrine glands throughout the body.

The Autonomic Nervous System

The autonomic nervous system, consisting of the sympathetic and parasympathetic nervous systems, is activated through complex processing at all levels of the central nervous system. The homeostatic control systems of the central nervous system often exert regulatory control over a wide variety of biochemical and physiological functions through a combination of sympathetic- and parasympathetic- sympathetic-induced physiological and biochemical responses. The sympathetic response can be nearly instantaneous, particularly with the effects on the cardiovascular system.

The Sympathetic Nervous System

Sympathetic nerves release neurotransmitters to cardiac muscle and smooth muscle in the bronchial walls, intestinal tract walls, and blood vessel walls. The neurotransmitters generate a rapid response to environmental circumstances that require aggressive and highly energetic responses (fight-or-flight responses). The sympathetic effects in such circumstances include increased force of heart contractions, increased heart rate, increased blood pressure, redirection of the blood flow from the intestines to the skeletal muscles, suppression of peristalsis, and dilation of the bronchial airways.

The sympathetic system also innervates the adrenal medulla and can cause the release of epinephrine and norepinephrine into the bloodstream, which creates a maximal and persistent overall state of dynamic alertness and physiological readiness to engage in the pursuit of prey, engage in physical combat, or escape from life-threatening situations.

The Parasympathetic Nervous System

The parasympathetic nervous system innervates most of the same glands, cardiac muscle, and smooth muscle cells as the sympathetic system. However, the effects of the parasympathetic system are the opposite of the sympathetic effects in most cases. The parasympathetic system is predominately activated during periods when the body requires rest and regeneration and/or must digest food. Perhaps most importantly, the body requires a continuously adjusting balance between the sympathetic and parasympathetic states. This balancing act is referred to as the autonomic tone of the body and is essential for the continuous optimal performance of all body systems.

Protective Reflexes

A vital class of specialized nervous system functions is the protective reflex class of functions. Notably, other primitive reflexes (e.g., the Babinski reflex, the root reflex, and others) are rather complex. The simple protective reflexes, most notably the deep tendon reflexes, are extremely simple two- or three-neuron circuits completely outside the central nervous system.

These reflexes respond instantaneously to stimuli that represent potentially dangerous forces acting on the body. Examples include the instantaneous withdrawal of a body part from a hot surface. The deep tendon reflexes are usually involved in this type of reflex, but they are also crucial when the limbs and joints are experiencing possibly catastrophic mechanical forces. The deep tendon reflexes have mechanoreceptors that trigger impulses when a dangerous level of mechanical stress is detected. Then, the mechanoreceptor signal travels through one or two neurons and synapses on a skeletal muscle that contracts to counteract the forces threatening injury at a bone or joint region. As a specific example of a deep tendon reflex, the patellar tendon reflex is elicited by tapping the patellar tendon of the knee with a reflex hammer.

RESPIRATORY SYSTEM

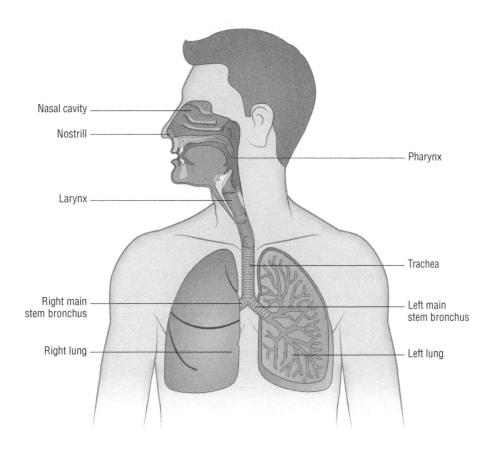

Nasal cavity

Nostrill

Pharynx

Larynx

Trachea

Right main stem bronchus

Left main stem bronchus

Right lung

Left lung

Root Word	Meaning	Examples
Rhin(o)-	nose	rhinitis, rhinorrhea (inflammation of and runny nose)
Laryng(o)-	larynx, voice box	laryngotomy, laryngectomy (cutting into, surgically removing the larynx)
Trache(o)-	trachea, "windpipe"	tracheotomy, tracheostomy (temporary and permanent openings)
Bronch(o)-	lung air passageways	bronchoscopy (looking into the bronchi)
Pne(u)-, -pnea	breath, air, lung	tachypnea, dyspnea, apnea (accelerated, difficult, painful cessation of breathing)
Pulmo-	lung	pulmonary artery
-ptysis	spitting (coughing)	hemoptysis (spitting or coughing up blood from lungs)
-plasty	reconstruction	rhinoplasty (surgical reconstruction of nose)

The Respiratory Tract

The initial segment of the respiratory tract is the trachea. The initial segment of the digestive tract is the esophagus. During swallowing, a specialized hinged plate structure (the epiglottis) can drop across the top of the trachea. This process prevents ingested solids and liquids from entering the trachea. The tracheal tube, which consists of rings of cartilage, descends through the anterior region of the neck (the trachea can be felt with one's fingers beneath the surface of the anterior neck). At the midpoint of the neck, a specialized region of the trachea (the larynx) can be seen and is commonly called the Adam's apple. The larynx contains the vocal cords and associated structures involved in the production of speech.

The trachea continues to the base of the neck and then enters the thoracic cavity. At about the mid-sternum level, the trachea bifurcates into a left and right main-stem bronchus. The right and left main-stem bronchi then enter their respective right and left lungs, then break into numerous subsequent and increasingly smaller branches and increasingly more air passages. These divisions result in a dense tree-like network of airways that infiltrate the entirety of the lung tissues. The thinnest terminal branches of this respiratory airway tree are called bronchioles. At the terminal ends of the bronchioles, grape-like clusters of spherical air sacs called alveoli serve as the site of oxygen and carbon dioxide exchange between the blood contained in capillaries encircling the alveoli and the inspired air in the alveoli.

The Respiratory System

Along with the respiratory tract anatomy already described, the respiratory system comprises the lungs, internal spaces of the thoracic cavity, and the muscular diaphragm that forms the thoracic cavity floor The lungs are composed of separate lobes, two on the left and three on the right. Positioned between the left and right lungs, the heart is directly adjacent to the medial surfaces of the left-lung lower lobe. Individual secondary bronchi branch off the main-stem bronchi and enter the lung lobes. The diaphragm is a dome-shaped muscle that is convex into the thoracic cavity. The superior surface of the diaphragm is adjacent to the inferior surfaces of the left and right lower lobes of the lungs. Importantly, the left and right phrenic nerves pass from the cervical spine through the center of the thoracic cavity and innervate the diaphragm. Damage to these nerves can paralyze the diaphragm, making the act of breathing impossible. The nasal sinuses also play a role in this system. These nasal sinuses are in cavities within the facial and occipital bones of the skull.

Respiratory Physiology

The primary functions of the respiratory system are to deliver oxygen from the air to the bloodstream and to remove carbon dioxide from the bloodstream into the air in the lungs and then out the body during expiration (exhalation). The primary tissues and structures of the respiratory system are the respiratory airway (trachea), bronchi and alveoli, the lung tissue, and the diaphragm. Breathing is usually involuntary but can be under voluntary control for short periods of time.

Nervous System Control of Respiration

The basal breathing rate is driven by the medulla oblongata. Peripheral sensory receptors in major arteries and veins and within the brain itself monitor oxygen and pH levels and report this information to the hypothalamus and the medulla. Breathing depth and rate is modified as necessary to maintain optimum levels of oxygen and blood PH.

The smooth muscle cells in bronchial airways are also innervated by the sympathetic and parasympathetic nervous system. Sympathetic signals cause relaxation of bronchial smooth muscle, which results in dilation of the bronchial airways. Parasympathetic signals have the opposite effect.

There is also a protective gag reflex that functions at the epiglottic region to prevent inhalation of solids or liquids.

Cilia

The epithelial cells lining the bronchial airways secrete mucous, and have numerous densely packed cilia, which have tiny, hair-like structures. The cilia on the bronchial airway membranes are in constant coordinated motion to propel mucus and inhaled particulate matter out of the lungs through the trachea, so the mucus can be more easily coughed up or swallowed.

Breathing Mechanics

When the epiglottis is open, the respiratory airways are continuous with the outside air. The flow of air is determined by the relative air pressures inside of the airway and the outside air. When the diaphragm contracts, the convex surface of the diaphragm within the thoracic cavity flattens; this increases the volume of the thoracic cavity surrounding the lungs, which causes a drop of pressure inside the thoracic cavity below that of the outside air. The resulting pressure differential between the airways within the lungs and the outside air drives air from the outside through the respiratory airways and into the alveolar air sacs.

Inspiration

The Lung tissue expands during the inspiratory phase of the breathing cycle. The Lung tissue is elastic and the expansion that occurs during inspiration dynamically stretches lung tissue. This process requires energy in the form of muscular work that is done by the diaphragm to increase the volume of the thoracic cavity and to decrease the pressure in the thoracic cavity.

Expiration

When the diaphragm relaxes, the elastic tissue in the lungs relaxes to its normal level of relaxation. Air pressure within the lung then increases and exceeds that of the outside air. Air within the airways is then driven out of the lungs by the differences in pressure inside and outside of the lungs. This portion of the breathing cycle is called expiration. Expiration – in contrast to inspiration – is normally a passive process that does not require energy utilization by the body.

Gas Exchange – Diffusion

At the microscopic level, gas exchange between the bloodstream and the alveolar air is driven by diffusion. Diffusion is movement of particles from one region to another region that is driven by difference in the concentration of particles between the regions. The blood arriving at the capillaries surrounding the alveoli is pulmonary arterial blood – which is deoxygenated. The oxygen concentrations in this blood are much lower and the carbon dioxide concentrations are much higher than the air contained in nearby alveolar air sacs. The walls of the alveoli are extremely thin, which allows a fast rate of diffusion to reoxygenate the blood.

Microscopic Physiology

The microscopic physiology of the capillary/alveolar region provides the optimum possible conditions for diffusion to occur – very short diffusion distances with a minimum of physical barriers to the diffusion process. Oxygen molecules must diffuse through a one-cell thick alveolar wall then through a one-cell thick capillary wall and then through a cell membrane of a red blood cell. The reverse is true for carbon dioxide molecules, which are diffusing in the opposite direction

– from the blood and into the alveolar air sacs. In the red blood cell, oxygen molecules bind to hemoglobin molecules.

This process reoxygenates the capillary blood and rids the blood of carbon dioxide. This blood is then delivered back to the heart for recirculation throughout the body.

DIGESTIVE SYSTEM

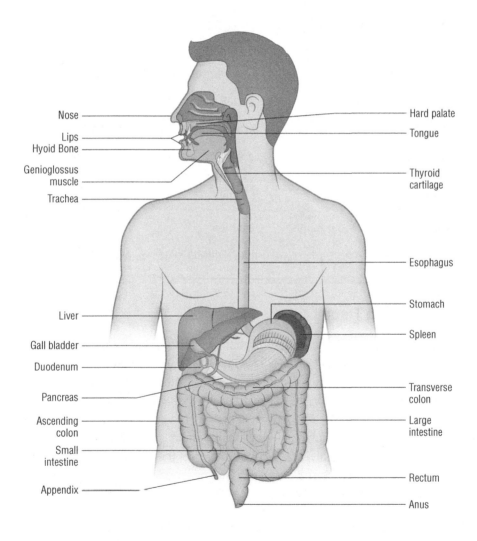

Nose

Lips

Hyoid Bone

Genioglossus muscle

Trachea

Liver

Gall bladder

Duodenum

Pancreas

Ascending colon

Small intestine

Appendix

Hard palate

Tongue

Thyroid cartilage

Esophagus

Stomach

Spleen

Transverse colon

Large intestine

Rectum

Anus

Root Word	Meaning	Examples
Gastr(o)-	stomach	gastritis, gastrectomy
Hepat(o)-	liver	hepatitis (inflammation of), hepatoma (tumor of)
Chol(e)-	gall, bile	cholecystitis, cholecystectomy (inflammation of, removal of gallbladder)
Cyst(o)-	bladder, sac	Cystoscopy (an endoscopy of the urinary bladder via the urethra)
Emes(o)-	vomit	emesis (vomiting), emetic (stimulating vomiting), antiemetic (stopping vomiting)
Lith(o)-	stone	cholelithotomy (removal of gallstones)
Lapar(o)-	abdominal wall	laparotomy (cutting into the abdomen)
-centesis	to puncture	abdominocentesis (puncturing and draining)
-tripsy	to crush	cholelithotripsy (smashing gallstones with sound waves)
-rrhea	flow, discharge	diarrhea
-iasis, -osis	abnormal condition	cholelithiasis (presence of gallstones causing symptoms)

The Digestive Tract

The digestive tract, beginning at the esophagus, follows along the same path as the trachea, immediately posterior or dorsal to the trachea. At the bifurcation of the trachea, the esophagus continues inferiorly to the base of the thoracic cavity, where it passes through an opening in the muscular diaphragm and enters the abdomen. Just after entering the abdomen, the esophagus connects to the stomach. A muscular sphincter—the gastroesophageal (GE) sphincter—seals the passage of the digestive tract at the junction of the esophagus and the stomach. The GE sphincter opens only during the passage of ingested material from the esophagus into the stomach.

At the distal end of the stomach, the digestive tract continues as the small intestine. The region of the small intestine that accepts the contents of the stomach is the duodenum. Another muscular sphincter (the pyloric sphincter) seals the passageway between the stomach and the duodenum. The sphincter opens at appropriate intervals to allow stomach contents to pass into the duodenum. In addition, substances produced by the liver and the pancreas that are involved in the digestive process are secreted into the duodenum through the common bile duct. The digestive process continues as nutrients and water keep moving through the small intestine, beginning at the duodenum and then passing through two subsequent segments of the small intestines, first the jejunum and then the ileum. The ileum connects to the first segment of the large intestine (the cecum).

At this point, all the nutrients and most of the water passing through the digestive tract have been absorbed. Indigestible bulk material continues to pass through the sequential segments of the large intestine, beginning with the cecum, and next the ascending, the transverse, and the descending colon. Most of the remaining water in the material within the large intestine is absorbed, and feces are formed during this stage through the digestive tract. The feces pass into the terminal segments of the large intestine (the sigmoid colon and the rectum) and then pass outside the body via defection through the anal sphincter.

The Digestive System

Along with the digestive tract anatomy already described, the digestive system also consists of salivary glands, the liver, the gallbladder, the pancreas, and a specialized regional venous circulatory system called the hepatic portal circulatory system. That system carries blood from capillary beds in the intestines to capillary beds in the liver. The salivary glands are in the oral cavity. The liver is on the right upper quadrant of the abdominal cavity, directly below the inferior surface of the diaphragm. The gallbladder is connected to the liver and nestled between liver lobes at the inferior surface of the liver. The pancreas is in the left upper quadrant of the abdomen, partially retroperitoneal (buried) in the dorsal abdominal wall.

The pancreatic duct and the gallbladder duct merge to form the common bile duct, which connects with the duodenum. An additional important anatomical relationship is that the stomach is anterior to the pancreas and inferior and to the left of the liver.

Digestive System Physiology

The function of the digestive system is to bring macronutrients, micronutrients, electrolytes, and water into the body. The macronutrients are carbohydrates, fats, and proteins. When dissolved in body fluids, electrolytes are the elemental ions Na+, K+, Ca++, Mg++, and Cl-. The micronutrients are vitamins and trace minerals. The digestive system also functions best when the diet includes indigestible plant fiber, which is composed primarily of cellulose.

An often-unappreciated fact regarding the digestive system is that, although the lumen (or canal) of the digestive tract is surrounded by the tissues and organs of the thorax and abdomen, the contents within the lumen of the digestive tract are literally outside the body. Nothing that has been consumed orally and is subsequently within the digestive lumen has been either absorbed by a cell of the body or passed through a surface epithelial cell layer into internal body regions.

The nutritional requirements of the body are the solid and liquid substances that must be consumed and then absorbed into the body. These substances include water, macronutrients, and micronutrients.

Peristaltic Motion

During swallowing, in the pharynx, the pulped food mass is compressed into a doughy consistency food-ball called a bolus. The bolus then passes into the esophagus. Beginning at the esophagus—and for the remaining journey through the digestive tract—the solid material in the food bolus will be propelled by rhythmic contractions of the digestive tract called peristalsis. This peristaltic motion is produced by smooth muscle cells in the walls of the digestive tract (esophagus, stomach, small intestines, and large intestines).

Intraluminal Barriers: The GE and Pyloric Sphincters

At the terminal (distal) portion of the esophagus, the food bolus must pass through a muscular sphincter. In biology, sphincters are rings of muscle tissue that can contract, just like the iris of the eye contracts, and thereby seal off a lumen (passageway), such as the lumen of the digestive tract. This process is called constriction; the relaxation of the sphincter reverses this action and opens the pathway, a process called dilation.

Normally, except when a food bolus is passing from the esophagus into the stomach, this sphincter—the gastroesophageal (GE) sphincter—is tightly constricted. This constriction occurs because the contents of the stomach are strongly acidic, roughly equivalent to the pH of battery acid. This stomach fluid will cause severe damage to any unprotected body tissues. When contents leak through the GE sphincter, heartburn occurs. A second muscular sphincter (the pyloric sphincter) is at the distal end of the stomach cavity, where the sphincter seals off the entryway to the initial segment of the small intestinal tract (the duodenum).

The Stomach

The stomach protects its inner wall lining from acidic injury by secreting large amounts of mucous onto the inner surface of the gastric lumen. To create this acidic environment, the stomach synthesizes and secretes hydrochloric acid. This highly acidic fluid by itself causes a widespread chemical breakdown of proteins and carbohydrates, but the stomach also synthesizes and secretes a powerful proteolytic (protein cutting) enzyme called pepsin. Pepsin is the first enzyme that engages in the enzymatic breakdown of all proteins.

Chyme

The stomach also engages is a considerable amount of mechanical digestion. The stomach walls are thick and constructed of several heavy muscle layers. This allows the stomach to generate powerful contractions that reduce food boluses into a slurry of water and partially digested lipids, proteins, and carbohydrates, collectively referred to as chyme.

The Small Intestine

At a time determined by the demands of the body, the stomach will release its contents into the adjacent distal segment of the digestive tract, the duodenum of the small intestine. The duodenum is the first of three continuous segments of the small intestine. The second segment is the jejunum, and the third and final segment is the ileum.

The Duodenum

The duodenum contains cells that synthesize and secrete the hormones secretin and cholecystokinin (CCK). Prior to stomach's releasing of its contents into the duodenum, these hormones are secreted into the bloodstream. The absorption of dietary iron occurs exclusively in the duodenum.

Bile

When arriving at the gallbladder, CCK stimulates the release of bile stored in the gallbladder into the gallbladder duct, which connects to the common bile duct. Bile then travels from the gallbladder duct into the common bile duct and then empties into the lumen of the duodenum. Bile that enters the duodenum is used to emulsify fats present in the digestive contents of the stomach once these contents are delivered into the duodenum.

REPRODUCTIVE SYSTEM

The male and female human reproductive systems are responsible for the generation of human offspring. The first stage of this process begins with the production of male and female gametes. Gametes, as a reminder, are the haploid (N) cells that result from meiotic cell division. In males, the gamete is a sperm cell; in females, the gamete is a mature ovum.

The second stage of this process is fertilization. During fertilization, male gametes are transported to the female reproductive system, and a sperm cell fuses with an ovum to produce a diploid (2N) cell, a zygote. The zygote is a hybrid cell that contains the following from the sperm cell and the ovum:

- **From the sperm cell:** one set of chromosomes 1 through 22 (the human autosomal chromosomes); one sex chromosome, which is either an X or Y chromosome.
- **From the ovum:** one set of chromosomes 1 through 22 and one X sex chromosome.

The resultant zygote has a full set of 22 pairs of autosomes and one pair of sex chromosomes (XX or XY). Zygotes with an X and a Y chromosome develop into male human offspring, and those with two X chromosomes develop into female offspring.

The zygote then begins the process of cell division and cell differentiation, which eventually leads to the production of a mature human fetus capable of independent survival outside the female reproductive system. At this stage, the fetus is born from the mother to the outside world through the process of labor and delivery.

The synthesis and secretion of the sex hormones—testosterone in the male and estrogen in the female—also occur in the gonads of the reproductive system.

Female Reproductive System

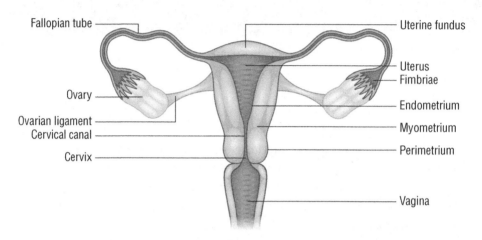

Root Word	Meaning	Examples
Hyster(o)-, metr(o)-	uterus	hysterectomy, endometritis (inflammation of the lining of uterus)
Salping(o)-, -salpinx	uterine tube	salpingitis, hematosalpinx (blood in the uterine tube)
Colp(o)-	vagina	colporrhaphy (suturing a tear), colpoplasty (surgical reconstruction), colposcopy (viewing the interior)
Oophor(o)-	ovary	oophorectomy, oophoropexy (surgery fixation, reattachment)
Men(o)-	menstruation	menarche (first), dysmenorrhea (painful menstruation)
Mamm(o)-, Mast(o)-	breast	mammogram, mastectomy
-pareunia, -coitus	intercourse	dyspareunia (painful intercourse), precoital (before intercourse), postcoital (after intercourse)

The female reproductive system consists of the external and internal female genitalia. The functions of the female reproductive system are the production of female gametes; the support of the fertilization of the fusion of female and male gametes to create a human zygote; and the physical support, protection, and nourishment of the development of the zygote to a mature human fetus and the subsequent delivery of the fetus to the outside world. The gonads of the female reproductive system are also responsible for the synthesis and release of the female sex hormone estrogen.

The External Female Genitalia

The external female genitalia, as a group, are called the vulva. The vulva consists of the mons pubis, which is a mound of fatty tissue overlying the pubic bone that forms the anterior segment of the vulva. The mons pubis comprises the labia majora, which are outer folds or lips divided into right and left labia by the pudendal cleft. The two folds of the labia majora are lateral to the underlying labia minora, clitoris, vaginal introitus (external opening), urethral meatus, the greater and lesser vestibular glands (Bartholin's glands and Skene's glands), and the vulvar vestibule.

The labia minora are similar in structure to the labia majora, are laterally located adjacent and inferomedial to the labia majora, and are adjacent and lateral to the central regions of the vulva. The central vulvar regions include the midline superiorly located clitoris and the centrally located vulvar vestibule. The urethral meatus and the vaginal introitus or orifice is in the midline of the vulvar vestibule. The urethral meatus is located immediately superior to the vaginal orifice.

The greater vestibular glands (Bartholin's glands) and the lesser vestibular glands (Skene's glands) are located lateral to the vaginal orifice. The Bartholin's glands secrete mucous that provides lubrication of the vagina and the surrounding vestibular regions.

The Female Internal Reproductive System

The female internal reproductive system consists of four major components: the vagina, the uterus, the fallopian tubes, and the ovaries. In contrast to the male reproductive system, the female urethra does not communicate with any female reproductive structures and has no role in the female reproductive system.

The Vagina

The vagina is an anatomical tube consisting of muscular and fibrous tissue. The lumen of the vagina begins at the vaginal orifice and extends internally to the pelvic cavity, where it terminates at the cervix of the uterus. The cervix is the inferior portion of the uterus and protrudes into the lumen of the vagina. The walls of the vagina encircle the cervix, and the interior lining of the vaginal lumen is continuous with the external surfaces of the cervix.

The Uterus

The functions of the uterus are (1) to serve as a site for the implantation of a developing embryo and (2) to provide a continuous supportive, nurturing, and protective environment for the continued development of the embryo into a viable human fetus. When the fetus is sufficiently developed to survive outside the uterus, the uterus undergoes a series of muscular contractions that expel the fetus from the internal uterine cavity through the cervical canal and into the lumen of the vagina.

The uterus is a pear-shaped muscular organ in the pelvic cavity in a position immediately adjacent and dorsal to the urinary bladder and immediately adjacent and ventral to the rectum. The uterus has four major anatomical regions: the cervix (neck of uterus), the internal os, the corpus (body of uterus), and the fundus (superior region of uterus). The conically shaped inferior segment of the uterus, the cervix extends into the vagina, forming the cap to the internal end of the vagina. In the central cervix region, a passageway continuous with the lumen of the vagina extends into the central cavity of the uterus.

The walls of the uterus consist of three layers. The innermost layer, which includes the internal surface of the central uterine cavity, is the endometrium. The endometrium includes an innermost epithelial layer, which in turn consists of a basal layer and an overlying functional layer. The functional layer includes the surface layer cells exposed as the lining of the central uterine cavity. The functional layer consists of epithelial cells, mucous glands, and blood vessels that are responsive to various hormones.

The functional layer undergoes an approximately once-per-month cycle of growth, degeneration, and regeneration (menstrual cycle) that occurs in response to the variations in the levels of hormones that regulate the menstrual cycle. The middle layer of the uterus is called the myometrium. The myometrium is composed of several thick layers of smooth muscle tissue. The outermost encapsulating layer of the uterus (the parametrium) consists of a continuation of the peritoneum, which is the epithelial surface layer of the abdominal cavity. The uterus is structurally supported in its position within the pelvic cavity by three pairs of suspensory ligaments: the uterosacral, cardinal, and round ligaments.

The Fallopian Tubes

The fallopian tubes are a pair of structures that extend from superior-lateral positions on the uterus, one on the left and one on the right, medial to a position directly opposite of the respective left or right ovary. The fallopian tubes contain a central lumen lined with ciliated epithelium. One end of the lumen is continuous with the central cavity of the uterus, and the other end is open to the pelvic cavity and faces the respective ovary. A short gap exists between the ovary and the lateral opening of the lumen of the fallopian tube.

During ovulation, when a mature follicle within the ovary ruptures and releases a mature ovum (female gamete), the ovum is drawn into the fallopian tube by local peritoneal fluid currents generated by the motion of cilia within the fallopian tube. Once inside the tube, the ovum is carried by the same ciliary motions into the central cavity of the uterus. Fertilization of the ovum by a sperm cell (which sometimes occurs within the fallopian tubes) triggers a set of reactions that allow the developing embryo to implant within the wall of the endometrium of the uterus.

The Ovaries

The ovaries are the female gonads. Ovaries are 3 to 4 cm in size and ovoid shaped. Two ovaries are present in females, one each in the pelvic cavity on either the left or right side just medial to

distal end of the respective left or right fallopian tube. The ovaries are connected to the uterus by the ovarian ligament and to the peritoneal wall of the pelvis by another ligament called the suspensory ligament.

In addition to being the primary estrogen-producing glands, the ovaries are organs that contain all a female's germ cells that will eventually mature and be released by the ovaries during ovulatory cycles. All these progenitor germ cells are present at birth in a human female's ovaries.

The general structure of an ovary includes an outer region called the cortex and an inner region called the medulla. The medulla of the ovary contains loose connective tissue that surrounds the blood vessels that provide the blood supply to the ovary.

The Ovarian Cortex

The ovarian cortex is composed of dense connective tissue, including fibroblast cells that can change functionally in response to various hormone levels. The cortex also has an outer layer of cuboidal epithelial cells called the germinal layer. While maturing into functional gametes (eggs), female germ cells acquire an organized collection of cells called granulosa cells. The granulosa cell mass and the embedded germ cell together are called an ovarian follicle. At all stages of development, the ovarian follicles are in the ovarian cortex.

Male Reproductive System

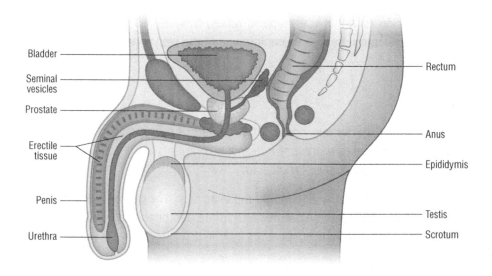

Root Word	Meaning	Examples
Orchid(o)-, Test(o)-	testes (male gonad)	orchiditis, orchidectomy, testicular artery, testosterone (male sex hormone)
Balan(o)-	head of the penis	balanitis
Andr(o)-	male	androgenic (stimulating maleness), androgynous (characteristics of male and female appearance)
Prostat(o)-	prostate	prostatitis, prostatectomy
Vas(o)-	vessel, duct	vas deferens, vasectomy (duct carrying semen from testes, cutting the duct)
-rrhaphy	to suture	herniorrhaphy (surgical correction of inguinal hernia)

The male reproductive system consists of the external male genitalia (the penis, the scrotum, and the testis) and the internal male genitalia (the distal segment of the urethra, the seminal vesicles, and the prostate gland, bulbourethral glands, and Cowper's gland). The penis consists of a central canal (the urethra) that also serves as the passageway for the delivery of urine from the bladder to the exterior of the body, and the distensible surrounding erectile tissue (the corpus cavernosum). The distal end of the penis forms the head or glans of the penis, which contain the external opening of the urethra (the meatus and surrounding tissue called the foreskin).

The scrotum, an external anatomical pouch or sack consisting of skin and smooth muscle, is divided into two chambers. Each chamber contains a single testis along with the associated structures of the testis (the epididymis and the ductus deferens). The scrotum allows the testis to experience a slightly lower temperature environment than the internal body temperature. This lower temperature environment is necessary to allow the proper functioning of the spermatogenesis (sperm production) that occurs within the testis.

The testes are ovoid-shaped organs responsible for the first stages of the production of sperm cells. The testes are enclosed by a tough outer membrane (the tunica albuginea). The interior of the testis consists of a collection of thin coiled tubules called the seminiferous tubules. The cells lining the interior of the semi-niferous tubules include specialized epithelial cells called Sertoli cells and germ cells capable of undergoing cell division and differentiation to produce sperm cells (spermatozoa).

The seminiferous tubules connect proximally to the rete testis, which is a short stalk of common connecting tubules where developing sperm cells are concen-trated before proceeding to efferent ducts and into the epididymis. The epidid-ymis is a highly convoluted tubule that forms a mass at the superior surface of the testis. Developing sperm cells are retained within the epididymis for 2–3 months. During this time, the developing sperm cell reach maturity.

The distal end of the epididymis is continuous with the vas deferens, which are short-length segments of tubules that connect the epididymis to the ejaculatory ducts in the interior of the pelvic cavity. The ejaculatory ducts connect to the urethra and have connections with ducts of the prostate gland, the bulbourethral glands, and Cowper's glands. These glands provide contributions to the seminal fluid that serves as the fluid medium that nourishes and supports the transpor-tation of sperm cells during ejaculation.

URINARY SYSTEM

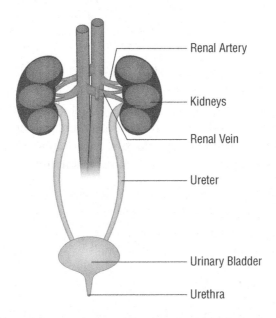

Renal Artery

Kidneys

Renal Vein

Ureter

Urinary Bladder

Urethra

Root Word	Meaning	Examples
Nephr(o)-, Ren(o)-	kidney	nephritis, renal artery
Hydro(o)-	water	hydronephrosis (abnormal condition involving back up of urine into the kidney
Cyst(o)-	bladder	cystitis, cystectomy (inflammation/ removal of bladder)

(Continued)

Root Word	Meaning	Examples
Pyel(o)-	renal collecting ducts	pyelogram (x-ray of the collecting ducts)
Ur(o)-, -uria	urine	polyuria, anuria (failure of the kidneys to produce urine)
Olig(o)-	scanty, less than normal	oliguria (reduced urine formation)
-pexy	to surgically reattach, fix in normal position	nephropexy (surgically attach kidney in normal anatomical position)

The urinary system consists of the kidneys, renal arteries and veins ("renal" is an adjective meaning related to the kidney or of the kidney), ureters, urinary bladder, and urethra. The kidneys are bean-shaped and located, as previously mentioned, within the walls of the abdomen in a dorsolateral position on either side of the lumbar spine. This "buried in abdominal wall tissue" location is referred to as a retroperitoneal position (the pancreas is also in a partial retroperitoneal position).

The renal arteries carry blood to the kidney that eventually arrives at capillaries surrounding microscopic filtering units called nephrons. Blood filtration occurs at these sites. Filtered blood from nephrons moves through venous networks and emerges from the kidneys within the renal vein. Filtered products from the nephrons pass through tubules that empty into a central collecting cavity in the kidney known as the renal pelvis.

The ureters (one per kidney) are thin tubes connecting the renal pelvis to the urinary bladder. The ureters transport the kidney's filtered liquid wastes (i.e., urine) from the renal pelvis to the urinary bladder. The urinary bladder is a distensible (inflatable) bag-like structure in the central anterior pelvic region of the abdominal/pelvic cavity. The bladder stores urine until it is released through another tube, the urethra.

The urethra carries the urine outside the body, exiting at the meatus (outer opening) of the glans penis in males and immediately anterior the entrance of the vagina in females. An additional important anatomical relationship of the urinary system is that the adrenal glands, which secrete many essential hormones as part of the endocrine system, are located directly adjacent to the superior surfaces of the kidneys, one adrenal gland per kidney.

The Kidneys

The kidneys have several critical functions in the human body. While kidneys produce urine, that is only the final stage of kidney function. The production of urine and its transport to the urinary bladder is the excretory function of the kidneys. This excretory function reflects the other functions of the kidney, which include maintaining an optimum volume of total body water and optimum concentrations of electrolytes within the fluid compartments of the body.

Additionally, the kidneys play a crucial role in maintaining an optimal pH of body fluids and in maintaining an optimum blood pressure. The kidney removes soluble waste products from the body, most notably urea, bilirubin, and organic acids, including uric acid and ammonia. The kidneys also have direct endocrine functions via the production of the hormones renin, erythropoietin, and calcitriol.

Gross Anatomy

There are two kidneys, each located anteriorly and laterally (either the left or right) of the spine in a retroperitoneal (buried in abdominal wall) position in the posterior wall of the abdominal cavity. Both kidneys are immediately inferior to the diaphragm. The left kidney is adjacent and posterior to the spleen. The right kidney is adjacent and posterior to the liver. The adult human kidneys are bean-shaped organs with an average size of about 10–13 cm in length, 5–7.5 cm in width, and 2–2.5 cm in thickness. The long axis of a kidney parallels the long axis of the body.

The lateral surfaces of the kidneys have a convex curvature, and the medial surfaces have a concave curvature. The upper region of the kidney is called the superior pole, and the lower region is called the inferior pole. In each kidney, an adrenal gland is located adherent to the superior pole.

Each kidney's outer surface is enclosed by a tough fibrous layer of tissue called the renal capsule. A layer of fat called the perinephric fat surrounds the renal capsule. The perinephric fat is surrounded by a connective tissue membrane called the renal fascia, which is surrounded by a second layer of fat (the paranephric fat layer). The renal hilum is a recessed region in the center of the medial surface of the kidney. The hilum contains the major blood vessels that supply the kidney (the renal artery and two renal veins) and the proximal end of the ureter.

The solid tissue of the kidneys is divided into two anatomical regions. The outer region is the renal cortex; the inner region is the renal medulla. The kidney is also subdivided into 10–15 renal lobes. The lobes are arranged sequentially like the wedges of an orange to produce the overall kidney structure. Each lobe consists of an upper or outer layer of renal cortex and a medial or deep cone-shaped region of renal medulla called a renal pyramid. The apex of each renal pyramid is called a papilla. Several adjacent renal papillae project into a cavity called a minor calyx. Several adjacent minor calyxes fuse medially into a larger cavity called a major calyx. The major calyces empty into a central cavity called the renal pelvis, which narrows into a tube that becomes the ureter. The ureter exits the kidney through the renal hilum and continues inferiorly to merge with the urinary bladder. Collectively, the renal pelvis and the major and minor calyxes form a continuous cavity called the renal sinus.

INTEGUMENTARY SYSTEM

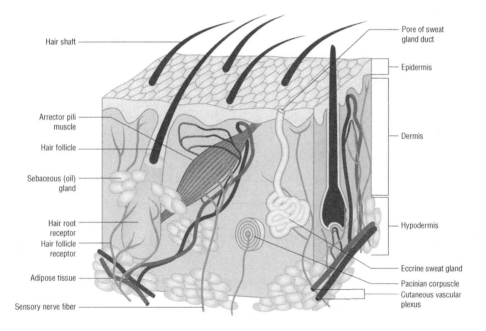

Hair shaft

Arrector pili muscle

Hair follicle

Sebaceous (oil) gland

Hair root receptor

Hair follicle receptor

Adipose tissue

Sensory nerve fiber

Pore of sweat gland duct

Epidermis

Dermis

Hypodermis

Eccrine sweat gland

Pacinian corpuscle

Cutaneous vascular plexus

Root Word	Meaning	Examples
Aden-	of or relating to a gland	adenocarcinoma, adenology, adenotome, adenotyphus
Adip-	of or relating to fat or fatty tissue	adipocyte
Carcin-	cancer	carcinoma
Cutane-	skin	subcutaneous
Dermat(o)-, Derm(o)-	of or pertaining to the skin	dermatology, epidermis, hypodermic, xeroderma
Dia-	through, during, across	dialysis
Hidr(o)-	sweat	hyperhidrosis
Hist(o)-, Histio-	tissue	histology
Leuc(o)-, Leuk(o)-	denoting a white color	leukocyte
Kerat-	cornea (eye or skin)	keratoscope
Lip(o)-	fat	liposuction
Onco-	tumor, bulk, volume	oncology
Onycho-	of or pertaining to the nail (of a finger or toe)	onychophagy
Papill-	of or pertaining to the nipple (of the chest/breast)	papillitis
Psor-	itchings	psoriasis
Py-	pus	pyometra
Sarco-	muscular, flesh-like	sarcoma, sarcoidosis
Squamos(o)-	denoting something as full of scales or scaly	squamous cell

Integumentary System

Root Word	Meaning	Examples
Trich(i)-, Trichia-, Trich(o)-	of or pertaining to hair, hair-like texture	trichocyst
Xer(o)-	dry, desert-like	xerostomia, xeroderma

The integumentary system of the human body, or simply "the integument," is a multilayered sheath of tissues and associated cells and extracellular structural and functional components that completely encloses the interior of the body. The most superficial layer of the integumentary system is exposed to the external environment and forms the external surface of the body. Two of the most general primary functions of the integumentary system are (1) to provide a physical containment of the internal body contents and (2) to provide a physical and biochemical barrier to elements of the external environment. Several secondary functions of the integumentary system exist as well. Most of these functions, as a group, can be categorized as homeostatic functions in the sense that they all provide mechanisms to maintain a controlled and stable, yet adaptable internal environment that remains distinctly separate from the external environment.

Layers of the Integument

The integument consists of a dermal or cutaneous layer and a subcutaneous or hypodermal layer. The dermal layer consists of two sub layers, the dermis and the epidermis.

The Hypodermis (Subcutaneous Layer)

As the lowermost or deepest layer of the integument, the hypodermis (subcutaneous layer of the integument) consists primarily of loose adipose connective tissue, blood vessels, lymphatic vessels, and nerves. The hypodermis provides a transitional connective zone between the overlying dermal layer and the adjacent underlying body contents, usually outer skeletal muscle layers, but in some areas, bony structures. Such structures particularly include those over the knee and elbow joints and the anterior surfaces of the lower leg (the shins).

The adipocytes of the hypodermis are organized into small collections called lobules that are enmeshed in collagen fibers. Fibroblasts are sparsely distributed throughout the hypodermis. The hypodermis-dermis boundary is a continuous series of interdigitating invaginations of both layers into the other with direct structural connections provided by collagen and elastic fibers. One of the four major types of mechanoreceptors—lamellar or Pacinian corpuscles—are located at the boundary region between the hypodermis and the dermis. These sensory receptor cells provide tactile information that results in the perception of pressure or vibration.

The Dermis

As the middle layer of the three major integument layers, the dermis is composed of three primary cell types (fibroblasts, macrophages, and adipocytes), but numerous other types of cells are interspersed within the dermis. Those cell types include chromophores or melanocytes and various cells associated with the immune system, including dendritic cells and T-cells.

The extracellular matrix of the dermal layers contain collagen, elastin, and reticulin fibers and several types of macromolecules that help to both retain water within the matrix and serve other functions. The most common types of these extracellular macromolecules are glycosaminoglycans, proteoglycans, and glycoproteins.

The Dermal Reticular Layer

The dermis consists of two sub-layers: the papillary layer, which is the superficial area adjacent to the epidermis; and the reticular dermis, which is a deep thicker area beneath the papillary layer. The reticular layer is composed of dense connective tissue that contains dense amounts of collagen fibers, elastic fibers, and reticular fibers. These fibers provide the mechanical properties of tensile strength and elasticity to the integument. The roots of hair follicles, sweat glands, sebaceous glands, and sensory receptor cells are also implanted within the reticular layer of the dermis.

The Dermal Papillary Layer

The papillary layer is immediately superficial to the reticular layer. The primary type of tissue contained in the papillary layer is areolar connective tissue. Areolar connective tissue is a very loose arrangement of adipocytes, and collagen and elastin fiber with an abundance of gel-like extracellular matrix. These features allow substances to readily diffuse through the tissue.

The Dermal-Epidermal Interface

At the interface between the papillary layer of the dermis and the overlying superficial layer of the integument (i.e., the epidermis), the papillary layer projects numerous knob-like extensions of tissue called papillae between interdigitating ridges of the epidermis, called rete ridges. The result is a tight enjoining of the two integumentary layers. The papillae of the papillary layer contain tufts of capillaries or Meissner's corpuscles, which are sensory receptor cells adapted to provide information interpreted in the central nervous system as the sensation of light touch. Mid portions of hair follicles, sweat and sebaceous glands nerves, and lymphatic vessels also travel through the papillary dermis toward the epidermis.

The Epidermis

The most superficial layer of the integument is the epidermis. The epidermis has no direct blood supply and depends on diffusion for the supply of oxygen and nutrients and for transport of CO_2 and other waste products. The epidermis begins immediately adjacent at the superficial surface of the papillary layer of the dermis. The two layers are separated by a basement membrane, which is a common feature of almost all epithelial tissues, serves as an attachment surface for the lowermost layers of epithelial cells, and creates anchoring connections with loose connective tissue located beneath the basement membrane. The basement membrane of the epidermis provides the biomolecular features that allow the epidermis to adhere to the dermis. The basement membrane has several additional functions, including immune system functions and cellular repair functions. The basement membrane has a complex structure consisting of multiple layers of fibrous proteins, including anchoring collagen fibers, substrate adhesion molecules (SAMS) integrins, and several other types of macromolecules. The basement membrane is also the last line of defense against the spread of cancerous cells that originate within the epithelium.

Regions of the Epidermis

The epidermis is composed of either four or five stratified regions depending on the local anatomical areas where the epidermis is located. Most areas consist of four regions: the stratum basale, stratum spinosum, stratum granulare, and stratum corneum. The epidermis of the palms of the hands and the soles of the feet is known as "thick skin" because it has five epidermal regions and is referred to as thick skin. The additional region of thick skin is the stratum lucidum, which is interposed between the stratum spinosum and the stratum granulare.

The Malpighian Layer

The deepest layer of the epidermis is the Malpighian layer, which is subdivided into the stratum basale or inner basal layer and the overlying stratum spinosum layer.

The basal layer (stratum basale)

The basal layer is composed of columnar epithelial cells attached to the super-ficial surface of the underlying basement membrane by connective structures called hemidesmosomes. These cells are germinal epithelium that undergoes mitotic division to produce a continuous supply of cells that migrate toward the outer surface of the epithelium. While migrating, these cells undergo progressive stages of differentiation with varying characteristics that define the overlying regions of the epidermis. The basal layer also consists of melanocytes, Merkel cells, and associated cutaneous nerves and cells that participate in the inflam-mation reactions of the immune system. Melanocytes connect to keratinocytes and provide the pigment melanin to keratinocytes. Melanin provides a barrier to ultraviolet radiation and is the pigment that determines the degree of darkness for skin tone, which a component of human racial characterizations. Merkel's cells and associated cutaneous nerves provide sensory information associated with the perception of light touch.

The stratum spinosum (spinous or prickle cell region)

The stratum spinosum is the second of the two sub-layers of the Malpighian layer of the epidermis. The stratum spinosum region is located directly superficial to the inner basal layer. This region consists of polyhedral-shaped cells that are daughter cells of the basal epithelial progenitor cells. The stratum spinosum cells also undergo mitotic division contributing to the approximately five layers of epidermal cells within the region. The cells have a spiny or prickly appearance due to microfilament shortening within desmosomes that interconnect among the cells. The stratum spinosum cells synthesize large amounts of fibrillar proteins called cytokeratin, which aggregates within the cells to form tonofilaments.

Tonofilaments are assembled into desmosomes, which form tight junctions between the epidermal cells while continuing to differentiate and migrate toward the epidermal surface.As keratinocytes within the stratum spinosum continue to migrate upward and differentiate, the Golgi within the keratinocytes begin to produce lamellar bodies that contain a complex assortment of phosphor, glycosphingolipids, free fatty acids and enzymes that have antibiotic activity. These products will eventually participate in the formation of the complex extracellular matrix of the outer epidermal layers.

The Stratum Granulosum

The region of the epidermis adjacent and superficial to the stratum spinosum is the stratum granulosum. The region is three to four cells in thickness. The cells of the granular region have a high content of keratin granules that produce a granular microscopic appearance, hence the name "granulosum" for this layer. The cells of the stratum granulosum are classified as keratinocytes, which do not divide in contrast to the cells of the stratum basale and the stratum spinosum. While continuing to be displaced toward the outer surface of the epidermis, keratinocytes become progressively flatter and more tightly compacted. In the palms and soles of humans, the stratum lucidum is a two-to-three cell-thickness region of the epidermis, and is adjacent and superficial to the stratum granulosum.

The Stratum Corneum

The most superficial region of the epidermis is the 10–30 cell-layer stratum corneum. Keratinocytes proceed through the final stages of cell differentiation to become corneocytes while moving from the stratum spinosum or stratum lucidum region to the stratum corneum. Corneocytes have ejected their cell nucleus (mature red blood cells also eject their cell nuclei) and are enveloped in a keratin protein matrix that, in turn, is surrounded by stacked layers of lipid molecules. The keratin proteins are connected to the cytoskeleton of corneocytes by structures called corneodesmosomes. This interconnection of corneocytes through keratin-corneodesmosomes-cytoskeleton networks provides the exceptional mechanical durability of the epidermis.

Glands of the Integument

The integument contains a variety of glands, most notably apocrine and eccrine sweat glands and sebaceous or oil glands. All these glands are exocrine glands. Exocrine glands secrete substances through a glandular duct (tube) onto the surface of epithelial tissue, either on the surface of the skin or on the luminal surface of an epithelial-lined hollow organ (e.g., the small intestine). In contrast, endocrine glands secrete substances directly into the bloodstream or lymphatic system.

Holocrine, Apocrine, and Merocrine Glands

Glands are also categorized based on the way they secrete substances. Three general types of secretory processes exist: holocrine, merocrine, and apocrine. Holocrine secretion occurs through the disintegration of the secretory cells when the disintegration of holocrine glandular cells releases the secretory substances present in the cytoplasm of the cells. Sebaceous glands of the integument are holocrine glands. The fragments of disintegrated glandular cells are also constituents of the secretions of holocrine glands. Apocrine secretion occurs through a budding of a cell membrane segment that forms vesicles that contain the secretory substances of the gland. Apocrine sweat glands are one of the two types of sweat glands in the integument. The cell membrane segments that bud off apocrine glandular cells are constituents of apocrine secretions. Human mammary glands are also apocrine glands.

The cellular fragment components of both holocrine and apocrine glands can obstruct the ducts of the glands. Obstructed glandular ducts can result in the formation of abscesses of the gland. The contents of these abscesses may become infected by bacteria, resulting in acne and other types of localized infections within the integument.

Merocrine glands utilize exocytosis to secrete their glandular products. No disintegration or budding of cell membranes occurs in the secretory cells of merocrine glands. The exocrine glands of the pancreas and virtually all endocrine glands are merocrine glands. The second type of sweat glands found in the integument (the eccrine sweat glands) are merocrine glands.

Sebaceous (Oil) Glands

Sebaceous or oil glands are widely distributed within the integument except for the soles of the feet and the palms of the hands. Sebaceous glands have ducts that most commonly communicate with the spaces adjacent to hair shafts within hair follicles, but a small percentage open directly onto the external epidermal surface. The glandular cells are in the dermis, usually adjacent to a hair follicle. Sebaceous glands are holocrine glands that synthesize and secrete a substance called sebum, which is an oily or waxy substance consisting of triglycerides, lipid esters, and free fatty acids.

Sebum provides an oily medium that contributes to the composition of the sweat layer on the surface of the skin. The oily component of sweat extends the cooling effects of evaporative sweating and prevents dehydration by increasing the adherence of the sweat layer to the surface of the skin. The free fatty acids contained in sebum lower the pH of the skin surface to a range of 4.5–5.0, a level that strongly inhibits the growth of potentially harmful microorganisms. In addition to the indirect antimicrobial effect provided by the lowering of skin pH, free fatty acids in sebum also provide strong, direct antimicrobial activity. The production of sebum can be influenced by various hormone levels; for example, testosterone stimulates sebum production, and estrogen inhibits sebum production.

Eccrine Sweat Glands

Eccrine glands are merocrine glands and are by far the most numerous and widely distributed type of sweat glands. Eccrine sweat glands secrete a watery solution containing sodium and chloride ions. In addition, eccrine sweat contains bicarbonate ions, cytokines, immunoglobulins, and short-sequence polypeptides that have antimicrobial activity. The secretory cells of the glands are coiled deep in the dermis. Myoepithelial cells surround the secretory cells, and the contraction of these cells propels sweat solution through the eccrine duct and onto the skin surface. Eccrine sweat glands are innervated by autonomic nerve fibers that modulate sweat secretion in response to core body temperature levels and emotional stress (e.g., excitement or fear).

Apocrine Sweat Glands

The secretory cells and surrounding myoepithelial cells of apocrine sweat glands are in the dermis near the dermis-hypodermis interface. The duct of apocrine sweat glands—like those of most sebaceous glands—is usually located adjacent to hair shafts within hair follicles. But the distribution of apocrine sweat glands is limited to only a few regions on the surface of the body, primarily the axillae (armpits). The composition of apocrine sweat gland secretions differs significantly from eccrine sweat compositions.

Apocrine secretions have a high protein and carbohydrate content. Apocrine sweat combines with sebaceous gland secretions in hair shafts in the axillae, resulting in a cloudy viscous solution that clings to axillary hair and supports colonization by bacteria. Colonizing bacteria break down components of axillary sweat, and these breakdown products are responsible for the characteristic odor associated with the axillary regions.

Abnormalities of the Integument

Notable abnormalities (pathologies) of the integument include impetigo (a superficial staphylococcal bacterial infection) and cellulitis (a deep bacterial infection that extends into the hypodermis). Superficial viral infections are typically caused by papilloma virus (warts), but many generalized viral infections produce surface viral-containing vesicles, such as those associated with the herpes virus. Superficial tinea-species fungal infections cause the condition known as athlete's foot. Generalized viral and other infections often produce immune-related skin rashes, and many drug hypersensitivities also produce skin rashes and mild temporary blistering in the form of hives. In more serious cases, deep blistering and skin loss can occur with poison ivy reactions, severe drug sensitivity, and infectious and autoimmune reactions. Eczema is a common hereditary hypersensitivity reaction of the skin. Psoriasis is an often severe and debilitating condition resulting from excessive rates of cell division in the epidermis. Malignant melanoma is a particularly deadly and common cancer of melanocytes, usually related to excessive sun exposure. The resistance of the integument to infection is generally impaired by high levels of cortisol, which are often associated with prolonged periods of psychological stress.

ENDOCRINE SYSTEM

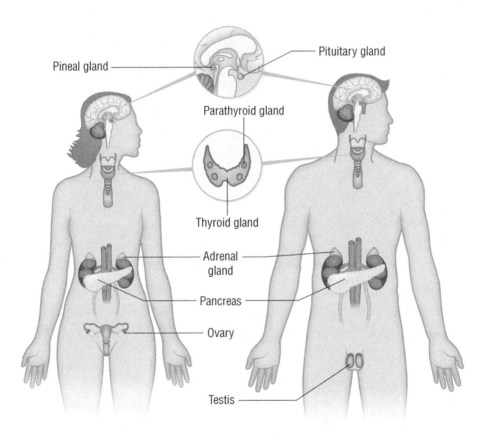

Pineal gland

Pituitary gland

Parathyroid gland

Thyroid gland

Adrenal gland

Pancreas

Ovary

Testis

Root Word	Meaning	Examples
Acr-	extremity, topmost	acrocrany, acromegaly, acroosteolysis, acroposthia
Aden-	of or relating to a gland	adenocarcinoma, adenology, adenotome, adenotyphus
Adren-	of or relating to the adrenal glands	adrenal artery
Andr-	pertaining to a man	android, andrology, androgen
-crine, Crin(o)-	to secrete	endocrine
-dipsia	(condition of) thirst	dipsomania hydroadipsia, oligodipsia, polydipsia
Eu-	true, good, well, new	eukaryote
Ex-	out of, away from	excision, except
Exo-	denoting something as outside another	exophthalmos, exoskeleton, exoplanet
Galact-	milk	galactorrhea, galaxy
Gluco-	sweet	glucocorticoid, glucose
Glyc-	sugar	glycolysis
Gon-	seed, semen; reproductive	gonorrhea
Home(o)-	similar	homeopathy
Hom(o)-	denoting something as the same as another or common	homosexuality, homozygote, homophobic
Hyper-	extreme or beyond normal	hypertension, hypertrichosis
Hyp(o)-	below normal	hypovolemia, hypoxia
Para-	alongside of	paracyesis
Somat(o), Somatico-	body, bodily	somatic

Root Word	Meaning	Examples
Thyr(o)-	thyroid	thyrotropin
Tox(i)-, Tox(o)-, Toxic(o)-	toxin, poison	toxoplasmosis

The endocrine system synthesizes and secretes hormones in the body. Hormones then exert a vast array of effects on the body. The endocrine system includes purely endocrine glands, whose sole function is the synthesis and secretion of hormones, and other tissues and organs that, in addition to their primary or co-functions, also synthesize and secrete hormones.

An important anatomical distinction exists between the two general types of glands, endocrine glands and exocrine glands. Exocrine glands do not necessarily secrete hormones and can secrete many other substances. The anatomical distinction for exocrine glands is that all exocrine glands secrete substances through a duct, which is a tube that leads to an anatomical surface (e.g., the surface of the skin or the surface of the intestinal tract). The common bile duct is one example.

All endocrine glands secrete hormones, and by anatomical definition, all endocrine glands secrete hormones directly into the bloodstream or the lymphatic system. In addition, by anatomical definition, no purely endocrine gland contains secretory ducts. For that reason, the endocrine glands are sometimes referred to as "ductless" glands.

The Hypothalamus and the Pituitary Gland

The hypothalamus and the pituitary gland are closely related anatomically. Together, these two structures serve as master controllers of the endocrine system through the secretion of hormones that regulate the levels of other hormones. The hypothalamus, a region of the brain that also synthesizes and secretes many critically important hormones, is in the inferior midbrain directly above the central region of the base of the cranial cavity. The pituitary gland is attached to the inferior portion of the hypothalamus by a connective stalk. The pituitary gland, which occupies a small depression or crater in the base of the skull called the sella turcica, secretes a wide variety of hormones. An Important anatomical feature of the pituitary gland is that the posterior pituitary synthesizes only two hormones—oxytocin and vasopressin—and all other pituitary hormones are synthesized by the anterior pituitary.

The Pineal Gland

The pineal gland is located within the midbrain and is essentially at the anatomical center of the brain. The gland produces melatonin, which regulates sleep patterns and circadian rhythms.

The Thyroid and Parathyroid Glands

The thyroid glands are located superficial and to either side of the midline of the tracheal cartilage. Many anatomists classify the thyroid as a single gland with left and right lobes. The parathyroid glands are notable for being, in a sense, glands within glands. Four parathyroid glands are typically buried deeply in the thyroid gland, usually two per lobe. The thyroid glands secrete thyroid hormones and calcitonin. The parathyroids secrete parathyroid hormone (PTH).

The Pancreas

The pancreas is not a purely endocrine gland. Despite serving a critical exocrine gland function as a part of the digestive system, the pancreas' endocrine function is even more important. The pancreas secretes the hormones glucagon and, most importantly, insulin. The pancreas, as previously described, is in the upper-right quadrant of the abdomen, in a partially retroperitoneal position, immediately below the diaphragm and posterior to the stomach.

The Adrenal Glands

As previously discussed, the adrenal glands rest upon the superior surface of the kidneys, one gland per kidney. The anatomical structure of the adrenal gland is significant in that the adrenal cortex (the surrounding outer layer) synthesizes the corticosteroid hormones, including cortisol and aldosterone, while the adrenal medulla (the central region) synthesizes epinephrine, norepinephrine, and dopamine.

The Gonads

The gonads have two important co-functions; the production of male or female gametes and the synthesis of sex hormones. In males, the gonads are the testicles and are located externally within the testicular pouches. The gonads synthesize the male sex hormone testosterone. In females, the gonads are the ovaries, which are located lateral to and at the level of the superior region of the uterus, one ovary on the left and one on the right. The distal entry into either the left or right fallopian tube is closely adjacent to the left or right ovary. The fallopian tubes provide a passageway into the uterine cavity. The uterus is a midline pelvic organ posterior to the urinary bladder and anterior to the rectum. The ovaries synthesize the female sex hormone estrogen.

Endocrine Physiology

While a large majority of the central nervous systems' responses are rapid in the form of electrical signals and muscular responses, the nervous system also exerts profound control over all aspects of the body through its influences on the endocrine system. In contrast to direct nervous-signal-mediated control, which generally produces rapid but short-lived effects, hormonal effects are usually much slower in their actions and are often cumulative over longer periods of time, in some cases years or even decades. Many hormonal systems also function relatively independently of the central nervous system. In addition, many other hormones or hormone-like molecules are produced and secreted by virtually all tissues and organs of the body. For instance, the duodenum synthesizes and secretes the locally active hormones CCK and secretin.

The Hypothalamic Hormones

The hypothalamus is a critical brain region for the maintenance of homeostasis within the body. A primary mode of this regulation of homeostasis by the hypothalamus is through the release of hypothalamic hormones. Below are the primary hormones secreted by the hypothalamus:

- **Thyrotropin releasing hormone (TRH)**: This hormone acts on the anterior segment of the pituitary gland and stimulates the release of thyroid-stimulating hormone (TSH).

- **Corticotropin-releasing hormone**: This hormone also acts on the anterior segment of the pituitary gland and stimulates the release of adrenocorticotropin hormone (ACTH)
- **Growth hormone releasing hormone (GHRH)**: This hormone stimulates the release of growth hormone (GH) from the anterior segment of the pituitary gland.
- **Gonadotropin-releasing hormone (GnRH)**: This hormone stimulates the release of follicle-stimulating hormone (FSH) from the anterior segment of the pituitary gland.
- **Somatostatin** (also known as growth-hormone-inhibiting hormone – GHIH): This hormone inhibits the release of growth hormone and follicle-stimulating hormone from the anterior segment of the pituitary gland.

The Pituitary Gland hormones

The pituitary gland is directly connected to the hypothalamus. Together, they regulate nearly all body functions via hormonal control. The two major functional/anatomical regions of the pituitary gland are the posterior pituitary and the anterior pituitary.

The Posterior Pituitary Gland Hormones

Many authorities consider the posterior pituitary to be part of the hypothalamus. The posterior pituitary secretes two hormones: oxytocin and vasopressin (also known as antidiuretic hormone – ADH).

Oxytocin

Oxytocin triggers the milk letdown reflex in nursing mothers.

Vasopressin (or ADH)

Vasopressin is a very important hormone that regulates blood pressure and the fluid balance of the body. The blood pressure effects are partially accomplished by ADH's effects on smooth muscle in the walls of blood vessels. ADH causes smooth muscle contraction in blood vessel walls, which in turn constricts blood vessel passageways. This results in an increase in blood pressure.

ADH also affects the microscopic filtering units of the kidney – the nephrons. There are an estimated one million nephrons per human kidney. ADH decreases the loss of water from the body by causing the nephrons to reabsorb water from fluids that have been filtered out of the bloodstream and are in the process of passing out of the kidney's filtering system and into the bladder.

Anterior Pituitary Gland Hormones

The hormones secreted by the anterior pituitary are described below.

Adrenocorticotropic hormone (ACTH)

ACTH is secreted continuously but at increased levels when the body is under physical or psychological stress and when blood glucose is too low. ACTH stimulates the cortex of the adrenal gland to release the corticosteroid hormone cortisol.

Thyroid-stimulating hormone (TSH)

TSH stimulates the thyroid gland to release thyroid hormones. Thyroid hormones are the primary hormones that establish the overall metabolic rates of the body.

Luteinizing hormone (LH) and Follicle-stimulating hormone (FSH)

LH and FSH are critical in the differentiation of cells to produce both male and female gametes and are the primary regulators of the female menstrual cycle.

Prolactin (PRL)

Prolactin stimulates glandular growth of mammary glands and subsequent production of milk in breastfeeding females.

Growth hormone (GH)

The levels of GH during childhood determines the maximum lean body mass and height that individuals can attain. This completion of growth is the physiological definition of adulthood.

Melanocyte-stimulating hormone (MSH)

The levels of MSH, particularly during prenatal (before birth) development, determines the darkness of skin color and is the basis for racial differences in skin color.

The Thyroid Hormones

The thyroid gland produces and releases two types of thyroid hormone, thyroxine (T4) and triiodothyronine (T3), and the hormone calcitonin. Notable effects of thyroid hormone include increases in the rates of protein synthesis, regulation of fat, protein and carbohydrate metabolism, promotion of cell differentiation, and enhancement of bone growth and regeneration. Excessively high or low levels of thyroid hormones can be fatal.

T3 and T4

Iodine atoms are included in the structure of the thyroid hormone and iodine deficiency leads to hypothyroidism and enlargement of the thyroid gland (this is called a goiter). The release of thyroid hormone is triggered by the pituitary hormone TSH. T3 is more potent than T4, but both hormones have the same effects. Thyroid hormones directly affect nearly every cell in the body and the overall effect is to increase the basal (baseline) metabolic activity of the body.

Calcitonin and Parathyroid Hormone (PTH)

PTH is synthesized and secreted by the parathyroid glands. PTH, along with the hormone calcitonin, is vitally important in the regulation of blood levels of calcium ion (Ca^{++}). The activity of calcitonin and PTH is on cells that are involved in the breakdown and regeneration of the calcium rich mineral hydroxyapatite—the major mineral that forms the extracellular matrix of bone.

The Pancreatic Hormones: Glucagon and Insulin

In addition to its exocrine function in the synthesis and release of digestive hormones and bicarbonate ions, the pancreas synthesizes and releases two hormones: glucagon and insulin. Both hormones are vital to maintaining proper levels of blood glucose. Insulin is also essential to most cells for the uptake of glucose into the cell. Insulin is produced by pancreatic islet cells. In type 1 diabetes, islet cells are attacked and destroyed by the body's own immune system. A lack of insulin can be fatal.

The Adrenal Cortical (Steroid) hormones – Cortisol and Aldosterone

The adrenal cortical hormones are steroid hormone. Steroid hormones are molecules that are modified versions of the cholesterol molecule. Other hormones are either small water-soluble molecules or polypeptides, which are amino acid chains.

Since the steroid hormones are based on a lipid type molecule, cholesterol, they are fat-soluble, rather than water-soluble. Steroid hormones are secreted into lymphatic vessels rather than blood vessels. The principal cortical hormones are the glucocorticoid steroid hormone cortisol, and mineral corticosteroid hormone aldosterone. The adrenal cortex also produces the precursor molecules that are transformed by the gonads into the male and female sex hormones, i.e., testosterone and estrogen.

Cortisol

Cortisol release is stimulated by the pituitary hormone ACTH. Cortisol has a wide range of actions including regulating the metabolism of fats, proteins, and carbohydrates. Cortisol also plays an important role in the immune system by suppressing the immune response. Cortisol also is involved in the regulation of glucose levels. Cortisol stimulates the liver to synthesize new glucose molecules through gluconeogenesis. Baseline levels of cortisol are essential to life.

Aldosterone

Aldosterone is a critical hormone in the regulation of blood pressure and electrolyte concentrations in the body. This regulation mechanism is highly complex and involves several other hormones in what is termed the renin-aldosterone-angiotensin hormone axis.

The Gonadal Hormones – Testosterone and Estrogen

The gonadal hormones—testosterone and estrogen—are synthesized in the testes in males and in the ovaries in females. The sex hormones are synthesized from cholesterol-based precursors that are produced in the adrenal cortex. During the prenatal stage, testosterone is responsible for the development of male external genitalia. During adolescence, the sex hormones are responsible for the development of secondary sexual characteristics—pubic hair, testicular maturation, and breast development. Estrogen also appears to provide protection from coronary artery disease and osteoporosis in premenopausal females.

IMMUNE AND LYMPHATIC SYSTEMS

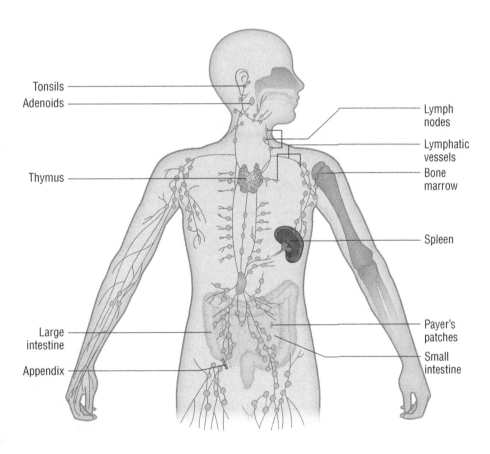

Tonsils

Adenoids

Thymus

Large intestine

Appendix

Lymph nodes

Lymphatic vessels

Bone marrow

Spleen

Payer's patches

Small intestine

Root Word	Meaning	Examples
Bas-	of or pertaining to base	basolateral
Blast-	germ or bud	blastomere
Cyt(o)-, -cyte	cell	cytokine, leukocyte, cytoplasm
Eosin(o)-	having a red color	eosinophil granulocyte
Hemat-, Haemato-, Haem-, Hem-	of or pertaining to blood	hematology, older form: haematolory
Hema-, Hemo-	blood	hemal, hemoglobin
Kary-	nucleus	eukaryote
Leuc(o)-, Leuk(o)-	denoting a white color	leukocyte
Lymph(o)-	lymph	lymphedema
Mon-	single	infectious mononucleosis
Morph-	form, shape	morphology
Phleb-	(blood) veins, a vein	phlebography, phlebotomy
-poiesis	production	hematopoiesis
Spleen(o)-	spleen	splenectomy
-stasis	stopping, standing	cytostasis, homeostasis
Thym-	emotions	dysthymia

The immune system is a complex and widely distributed network of cells, organs, and other structures, while the lymphatic system is a body-wide circulatory system that includes lymphatic vessels, lymph nodes, and lymphoid organs. The lymphatic vascular system is closely associated in both structure and distribution to the blood vessels of the cardiovascular system. The lymphatic system functions include the removal of excess fluids and debris from the extracellular or interstitial compartments of the body (the area surrounding cells, not including spaces inside blood vessels). The lymphatic system is also a major component of the immune system.

Capillary-size lymphatic vessels are found throughout the body. These vessels are terminal branches of the lymphatic vascular system. Lymphatic fluid moves from interstitial spaces into the lymphatic capillaries, then to progressively larger vessels, and finally to lymph nodes. Lymph nodes are nodular structures widely distributed throughout the body. Lymphatic fluid is filtered at lymph nodes and continues in vessels, leaving the lymph nodes to reach one of the two major lymphatic vessels—either the right lymphatic duct or the thoracic duct. The right lymphatic duct delivers lymph fluid into the right subclavian vein, and the thoracic duct delivers lymphatic fluid into the left subclavian vein.

The lymphatic circulation is also responsible for the absorption of fats and fat-soluble vitamins (vitamins A, C, D, and E) in the small intestines and subsequently for transport to the bloodstream.

Lymph Nodes

The anatomy of lymph nodes is significant for two key reasons: (1) the cortex of the lymph node is a site where T-cells accumulate and interact with B-cells, and (2) the medulla of lymph nodes is one of the anatomical regions where the maturation of B-cells occurs.

The Spleen

The spleen, the largest lymphoid organ in the body and one of the larger organs of the body in general, is in the left-upper quadrant of the abdomen just superior to the stomach and just inferior to the diaphragm. The spleen has structures that resemble lymph nodes containing B- and T-cells. It filters blood that arrives via the splenic artery arteries. The spleen contains macrophages that consume damaged and elderly red blood cells and recycles iron to the liver; and it also contains a large volume of white blood cells that serve as a readily accessible reserve for immune activities that may be required by the body.

The Thymus

The thymus is an organ in the midline of the thoracic cavity immediately posterior to the sternum and anterior to the trachea, directly between the lungs. The thymus is the organ where Tcells maturate.

The Appendix and the Tonsils

The appendix, and the tonsils are also lymphoid organs that contain B- and T-cell functional regions. The appendix is an appendage of the cecum of the large intestine. The tonsils are in the lateral walls of the pharynx.

Bone Marrow

The medulla (central region) of most skeletal bones—and particularly the long bones of the arms and legs and the pelvic bones—contain bone marrow. Both red blood cells and white blood cells (including immature T- and B-cells) are produced in bone marrow.

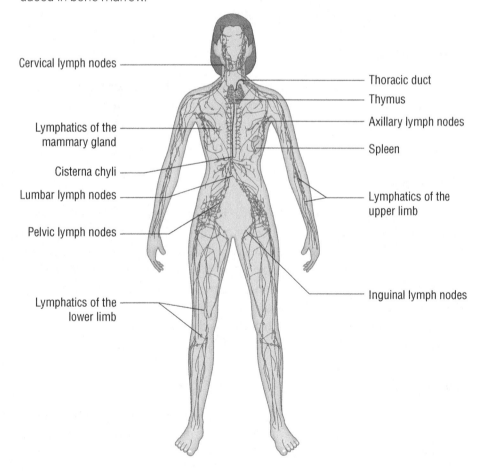

Cervical lymph nodes

Thoracic duct

Thymus

Lymphatics of the mammary gland

Axillary lymph nodes

Spleen

Cisterna chyli

Lumbar lymph nodes

Lymphatics of the upper limb

Pelvic lymph nodes

Lymphatics of the lower limb

Inguinal lymph nodes

Immune and Lymphatic Systems

Immune System Physiology

Most authorities would agree that the nervous system is probably the most complex system of the human body. At the same time, however, the human immune system is also extraordinarily complex, and decades of research remains to answer large gaps in the existing knowledge about this system. The immune system functions to protect the human body from foreign disease-causing biological and chemical agents. These agents include viruses, bacteria, and other single- and multi-cellular organisms. The immune system also protects the body from chemical products produced by disease-causing organisms such as toxins. Finally, the immune system attempts to identify and contain or destroy dysfunctional or cancerous cells of the body.

There are various ways to categorize the immune system, one is to define functions as either innate or adaptive immune system response.

Innate Immune system

The innate immune system is a non-specific or generic immune system. It responds to pathogens and to any other events that cause injuries to the body. In contrast to active immunity, innate immunity does not provide long-lasting resistance to repeated infection by the same organism.

Anatomical Barriers

The innate immune consists of anatomical barriers and a variety of chemicals and cell types. The skin provides a physical barrier to pathogens and rids the skin surface of pathogens by desquamation (skin flaking), by sweating, and by the production of organic acids that create an unfavorable skin pH for pathogens. The continuous transport of mucus out of the respiratory tract by the motion of cilia provides physiological barriers to pathogens in the respiratory tract. The peristaltic motion of the intestines transports pathogens out of the digestive tract and gastric, and bile acids and digestive enzymes create a very hostile environment to most living organisms. Those organisms that do thrive in the digestive tract create a bio community that resists intrusion of other organisms. Saliva, mucous and other bodily secretions contain a potent antibacterial compound called lysozyme.

Natural Killer Cells

If the barriers to a pathogen are breached, there are several innate defenses that are triggered. If the pathogen infects a cell of the body - usually in the form of a virus - the infected cell will alter its surface membrane molecules to alert natural killer (NK) cells that the cell is injured or infected. The NK cells attack the unhealthy cell by releasing perforins - small molecules that assemble on the target cell membrane and create holes or pores in the cell membrane. This can be sufficient to kill the cell but the NK cells also use the perorations created in the cell membrane to pass a potent toxin into the cell. The toxin has rapidly fatal effects on the unhealthy cell.

Sentinel Cells and Cytokines

Pathogens that are not confined to the interior of cell are identified by monitoring cells of the innate immune system. These are also called sentinel cells or surveillance cells. They recognize a limited number of molecular features common to most biological pathogens. As these pathogens enter the body, sentinel cells (usually macrophages) identify them and release molecules called cytokines.

Inflammation and the Complement Cascade

Cytokines are a class of intercellular signaling molecules that have a wide range of actions. One such reaction is the inflammatory reaction, which generates fever, vasodilation, and activates the complement cascade—a series of chemical reactions that produce large amount of protein products that can directly kill pathogens or can bind to pathogens and make them highly susceptible to destruction by macrophages.

Interferons

Interferons are a class of a number of specific molecules released by many cells that progressively restrict the ability of viruses to continue infectious cycles within the body.

Macrophages

Macrophages are cells of the immune system that literally consume other cells—pathogens and injured or dead cells of the body, a process called phagocytosis. Fever raises body temperature to levels that are unfavorable for viral infection processes. Swelling and increased blood flow begins the process of drawing a variety of types of immune cells to infection sites where an increasingly complex battle is waged to wall off the pathogens from further entry into the body and ultimately to kill the pathogens and then to remove the cellular debris that results from this immunological warfare.

Histamine

Another class of effects that greatly enhances the local inflammatory reactions is the triggering of the release of histamine—this molecule causes local pain, increases fluid leakage from blood vessels at the infection site, resulting in swelling and causing vasodilation that results in an increased blood flow to the infected region.

Neutrophils

Another class of cytokine effects is the attraction of large numbers of neutrophil, which is a type of leukocyte, to the site of the pathogenic infection. This process involves the production of intercellular adhesion molecules (ICAMs) that neutrophils recognize and follow to the infection site. Upon encountering pathogens, neutrophils release granules of highly toxic compounds that destroy the cellular invaders.

As the innate immune response proceeds, a large number of additional inflammatory chemicals are produced. Several other cell types arrive and begin to create an inflammatory exudate of proteins, cells, and cytotoxic chemicals at the site of infection. When successful, the infection is walled off, pathogens are destroyed, and the damages are repaired.

Adaptive Immune system

The adaptive immune system consists of two major types of white blood cells called lymphocytes. The two types of lymphocytes are T-cells and B-Cells. B-cells produce antibodies - which are incredibly specific molecules that are designed to bind to a small molecule or a small region of a larger molecule. These small molecular regions are called antigens. Antigens are chemically foreign to the body and are considered "non-self" elements that the adaptive immune system recognizes and subsequently attempt to remove or deactivate by producing the specific antibody to the antigen or by immune cell actions that directly kill a pathogenic cell.

Humoral Active Immune Responses

In the humoral adaptive immune response, B-cells produce circulating antibodies that bind to antigens anywhere in the body. Interactions between circulating antigens, B-cell, and T-helper cell (a subtype of T-cell) trigger B cells to proliferate and to produce large amounts of antibodies. When circulating antibodies bind these antigens, an antigen-antibody complex is formed, and this complex can be removed from the body by various mechanisms.

Cell-Mediated Active Immune Responses

The cell-mediated adaptive immune response involves the interaction of T-cells, B-cells, and antigen presenting cells or pathogen capturing cells in the form of macrophages. In one type of cell-mediated response a macrophage binds to a foreign cell, and then a T-helper cell binds to the macrophage. This binding action causes the T-helper cell to release cytokines that attract the cytotoxic T-cell to the T-helper/macrophage/pathogen cell complex. The cytotoxic T-cell, upon arrival, then kills the pathogenic cell.

Protective (Long-Term) Immunity

The innate immune system responds to pathogens and other substances that can injure cells (chemical, thermal and physically inflicted injuries) in the same way every time. The adaptive immune system provides protective immunity.

Once a particular antigen or pathogen has been identified by the adaptive immune system, the system is then primed to respond very quickly and very rapidly to clear the body of that particular antigen or pathogen if it attempts to infect the body in the future. This type of protective immunity can be artificially produced by the administration of vaccines. Typically, a vaccine is an injection of antigens in the form of killed or weakened pathogenic bacteria or viruses, which will result in long-term protective immunity to the native dangerous form of the bacterial or virus.

Passive Immunity

Passive immunity is a short-term immunity to pathogens that is acquired, rather than produced. For example, nursing infants acquire passive immunity to various pathogens by consuming antibodies formed by the mother and passed to the infant via breast milk. Once the supply of these antibodies stops, the immunity to the antibody-specific pathogens disappears in a few weeks or months.

MEDICAL ABBREVIATIONS

Just as important as knowing proper medical terminology is the ability to communicate that information effectively and efficiently in the real world. Typing and spelling out such long words would be neither efficient nor effective, so many abbreviations and acronyms are commonly used in writing notes and orders.

Below, the long list of medical abbreviations is broken up into relevant sections for easier use. The good news is that many of these abbreviations are for common English words. Still, readings an abbreviation in a list with the definition next to it is one thing, while having no "cheat sheet" to reference in the real world is quite another.

General Abbreviated Terms

Abbreviation	General Term
AA	amino acid
ABG	arterial blood gas
ADM	admission, admitted
ALS	advanced life support, amyotrophic lateral sclerosis
AMA	against medical advice, American Medical Association
ASAP	as soon as possible
A&W	alive and well

(Continued)

Abbreviation	General Term
c	centigrade, Celsius
cc	cubic centimeter, chief complaint, critical care, complications, carbon copy
C/O	complains of, care of
CO2	carbon dioxide
D/C	discontinue or discharge
DNR	do not resuscitate
DO	disorder
DOA	dead on arrival or date of admission
DOB	date of birth
DOT	directly observed therapy
DSM	Diagnostic and Statistical Manual of Mental Disorders
EDC	estimated date of confinement
EGA	estimated gestational age
ER	emergency room
F	Fahrenheit
H&P	history and physical examination
HPI	history of present illness
H/O	history of
HR	heart rate or hour
HS	hour of sleep (bedtime)
ICU	intensive care unit
ID	infectious diseases

Abbreviation	General Term
IP	inpatient
IQ	intelligence quotient
IU	international units
MCO	managed care organization
MG	milligram
MVA	motor vehicle accident
ML	milliliter
NKDA	no known drug allergies
NTG	nitroglycerin
O2	oxygen
OPD	outpatient department
P	pulse
Post op	postoperative (after surgery)
Pre op	preoperative (before surgery)
PA or PT	patient
PCP	primary care physician
RBC	red blood cell
RF	risk factor
s	without (sans)
sx	symptoms
s1s	signs and symptoms
STAT	immediately
T	temperature

(Continued)

Abbreviation	General Term
TPR	temperature, pulse, respiration
USOH	usual state of health
vs	vital signs
vss	vital signs stable
WB	whole blood
WBC	white blood cell
WNL	within normal limits

Prescription and Drug Abbreviations

Abbreviation	Prescription/Drug Term
ABX	antibiotics
AC	before meals
Ad lib	at will, as desired
BID	bis in dies (twice a day)
CAP	capsule
GTT	drop: liquid measurement
i	1
ii	2
iii	3
iv	4
v	5
MDD	maximum daily dose
NPO	nothing by mouth
OCP	oral contraceptive pill
OPV	oral polio vaccine
OTC	over the counter
PC	after meals
PCN	penicillin
PNV	prenatal vitamins
PO	per os (by mouth)
PRN	as needed
q2h	every 2 hours

(Continued)

Abbreviation	Prescription/Drug Term
q3h	every 3 hours
qam	every morning
qd	once a day
qh	once every hour
qhs	at bedtime
qid	four times a day
qod	every other day
qpm	every evening
RDI	recommended daily intake
Rx	prescription, treatment
SC/SQ	subcutaneous
TAB	tablet
TIW	three times a week

Care and Procedural Abbreviations

Abbreviation	Care and Procedural Term
AXR	abdominal x-ray
BAC	blood alcohol content
BC	birth control
BE	barium enema
BMT	bone marrow transplant
Bx	biopsy
BRP	bathroom privileges
CPR	cardiopulmonary resuscitation
CXR	chest x-ray
ECC	emergency cardiac care
ECG or EKG	electrocardiogram
ECMO	extracorporeal membrane oxygenation
ECT	electroconvulsive therapy
ECV	external cephalic version
FB	foreign body
FNA	fine needle aspiration
FOBT	fecal occult blood testing
GLT	glucose loading test
GTT	glucose tolerance test
H2O	water
I&D	incision and drainage
IM	intramuscular

(Continued)

Abbreviation	Care and Procedural Term
I&O	intake and output
IV	intravenous
IUPC	intrauterine pressure catheter
In vitro	in the laboratory
In vivo	in the body
KUB	kidney, ureter, bladder (x-ray)
OGTT	oral glucose tolerance test
PAP	pulmonary artery pressure; Papanicolaou test
PEEP	positive end expiratory pressure
PT	physical therapy
T&C	type and cross (blood)
TPA	tissue plasminogen activator (dissolve clots), total parenteral alimentation (intravenous nutritional needs)
UA	urinalysis
US	ultrasound
XRT	external radiation therapy

Patient Condition or Diagnoses Abbreviations

Abbreviation	Patient Condition/Diagnosis Term
ADHD	attention deficit hyperactivity disorder
AF	acid fast
AIDS	acquired immune deficiency syndrome
A&O	alert and oriented
AOB	alcohol on breath
ARDS	adult respiratory distress syndrome
ARF	acute renal failure, acute rheumatic fever
BAD	bipolar affective disorder
BM	bowel movement
BP	blood pressure
CA	cancer
CAB	carotid artery bruit
CABG	coronary artery bypass graft
CAD	coronary artery disease
CBC	complete blood count
CF	cystic fibrosis
C/F	chills, fever
CFT	complement fixation testing
CHD	congenital heart disease
CHF	congestive heart failure
COLD	chronic obstructive lung disease
COPD	chronic obstructive pulmonary disease

(Continued)

Abbreviation	Patient Condition/Diagnosis Term
CP	chest pain
CP	cerebral palsy
C/S	cesarean section
CV	cardiovascular
CVA	cerebral vascular accident (stroke)
DTR	deep tendon reflex
DVT	deep venous thrombosis
Dx	diagnosis
EBL	estimated blood loss
EBV	Epstein Barr virus
EC	eye contact
ECASA	enteric coated acetylsalicylic acid
EGC	early gastric cancer
FAS	fetal alcohol syndrome
FB	foreign body
F/C	fever, chills
FEF	forced expiratory flow
FHR	fetal heart rate
FM	fetal movement
FRC	functional residual capacity
FSE	fetal scalp electrode
FSH	follicle stimulating hormone
FT	full term

Abbreviation	Patient Condition/Diagnosis Term
FX	fracture
GA	gestational age
GH	growth hormone
GHRH	growth hormone releasing hormone
GI	gastrointestinal
GLT	glucose loading test
GSW	gunshot wound
GTT	glucose tolerance test
GU	genitourinary
HA	headache
HA	hemolytic anemia
HAV	hepatitis A virus
HBV	hepatitis B virus
Hb	hemoglobin
HCV	hepatitis C virus
HDL	high density lipoprotein
HDV	hepatitis D virus
HIV	human immunodeficiency virus
HPA	hypothalamic suppression test
HR	heart rate
HTN	hypertension
IBD	inflammatory bowel disease
IBS	inflammatory bowel syndrome

(Continued)

Abbreviation	Patient Condition/Diagnosis Term
ICP	intracranial pressure
IDDM	insulin dependent diabetes mellitus
IPF	idiopathic pulmonary fibrosis
IUI	intrauterine insemination
IUP	intrauterine pregnancy
IVF	in vitro fertilization
IVIG	intravenous immune globulin
IVP	intravenous push
JCV	JC virus
JRA	juvenile rheumatoid arthritis
JVD	jugular venous distension
KS	Kaposi sarcoma
LAD	leukocyte adhesion deficiency
LBP	lower back pain
LBW	low birth weight
LIH	left inguinal hernia
LOF	loss of fluid
MD	muscular dystrophy
MR	mental retardation
MS	multiple sclerosis
NAD	no acute distress
Nat/O	birth
NIDDM	non-insulin dependent diabetes mellitus

Medical Abbreviations

Abbreviation	Patient Condition/Diagnosis Term
NM	neuromuscular
N/V	nausea vomiting
NVD	normal vaginal delivery
OCD	obsessive compulsive disorder
ON	optic neuritis
OSA	obstructive sleep apnea
PD	Parkinson's disease
PE	pulmonary embolism
PKD	polycystic kidney disease
PID	pelvic inflammatory disease
PIH	pregnancy induced hypertension
PMS	premenstrual syndrome
PTSD	post-traumatic stress disorder
RA	rheumatoid arthritis
RAD	reactive airway disease
RDS	respiratory distress syndrome
REM	rapid eye movements
RHD	rheumatic heart disease
RXN	reaction
SAB	spontaneous abortion
SBO	small bowel obstruction
SBS	shaken baby syndrome
SOB	shortness of breath

(Continued)

Abbreviation	Patient Condition/Diagnosis Term
STD	sexually transmitted disease
TAH	total abdominal hysterectomy
TB	tuberculosis
TBI	traumatic brain injury
TGA	transient global amnesia
UC	ulcerative colitis
UO	urine output
URI	upper respiratory infection
UTI	urinary tract infection
VB	vaginal bleeding
VBAC	vaginal birth after cesarean section
VF	ventricular fibrillation
VH	vaginal hysterectomy, hallucination
VIP	voluntary interruption of pregnancy

Anatomical and Body Abbreviations

Abbreviation	Anatomical and Body Term
ABD	abdomen
AD	right ear
AL	left ear
AU	both ears
BMD	bone mass density
BMI	body mass index
BMR	basal metabolic rate
CBD	common bile duct
CBF	cerebral blood flow
FL	femur length
FROM	free range of motion
HC	head circumference
IBW	ideal body weight
LLL	left lower lobe
LLQ	left lower quadrant
LUL	left upper lobe
LUQ	left upper quadrant
LV	left ventricle
OD	right eye
OS	left eye
OU	both eyes
PNS	peripheral nervous system

(Continued)

Abbreviation	Anatomical and Body Term
RA	right atrium
RUL	right upper lobe
RUQ	right upper quadrant
RV	right ventricle, residual volume
TLC	total lung capacity
UE	upper extremity
WT	weight

Made in the USA
Coppell, TX
23 June 2024

33836308R00105